ILLUSTRATED CASE HISTORIES

Urology

Helen Parkhouse

Consultant Urologist
The Hillingdon Hospital
London, UK

Krishna Sethia

Consultant Urologist
Norfolk and Norwich Hospital
Norwich, UK

M Mosby-Wolfe
MEDICAL COMMUNICATIONS

Project Manager:	Jane Hurd-Cosgrave
Developmental Editor:	Lucy Hamilton
Production:	Mike Heath
Index:	Anita Reid
Publisher:	Geoff Greenwood

Copyright © 1995 Times Mirror International Publishers Limited.

Reprinted in 1996 by Mosby-Wolfe Medical Communications, an imprint of Times Mirror International Publishers Limited.

Originated in Mandarin Offset Ltd, Hong Kong.

Printed by Grafos S.A. Arte sobre papel, Barcelona, Spain.

ISBN 0 7234 2234 6

For full details of all Times Mirror International Publishers Limited titles, please write to Times Mirror International Publishers Limited, Lynton House, 7–12 Tavistock Square, London WC1H 9LB, England.

A CIP catalogue record for this book is available from the British Library.

Library of Congress Cataloging-in-Publication Data has been applied for.

Warning

The doses of pharmaceutical products given in this book are a guide only. Although every effort has been made to be accurate, the authors and publishers cannot be held responsible for the accuracy of these dosages. It is recommended that the reader, if in any doubt, checks in the latest editions of publications such as the British National Formulary, Martindale's Extra Pharmacopoeia or MIMS (Monthly Index of Medical Specialities).

Contents

Preface

The cases shown are all genuine cases seen by the authors over a number of years. The cases have been selected to be of interest to trainees in Urology and Radiology and to general practitioners who are being increasingly involved in the shared care of patients with urological problems.

As these are all individual case histories, the diagnostic pathways and the treatments described may not necessarily be applicable to other cases. Urology is a speciality which continues to evolve, largely as a result of new technology in diagnostic imaging and advances in therapy, so that the clinician now has considerable choice in the management of an individual patient. We do not claim to have included all management options, but hope to encourage further reading in current journals and comprehensive textbooks.

Acknowledgements

We are grateful to the following colleagues who have provided material for illustrations: Mr. M. H. Ashken, Dr. R. J. Ball, Dr. F. Barker, Mr. N. Burgess, Dr. N. Chetty, Mr. N. A. Green, Dr. M. Hall–Craggs, Dr. R. Kantor, Dr. J. Latham, Mr. H. Laing, Mr. N. Parkhouse, Mr. R. Persad, Dr. G. Rustin.

Case 1
A Boy Called "Smelly"

A nine-year-old boy was referred to the endocrinology clinic for investigations of short stature. During the course of investigations he was found to have chronic renal failure with a serum creatinine of 350 μmol/l, and on detailed questioning it was discovered that he was nicknamed "Smelly" at school because of his continual urinary and faecal incontinence. On examination he was found to have a deep cutaneous dimple overlying the sacrum, and the sacrum was only partially palpable.

QUESTIONS
1. What abnormalities are seen on plain abdominal radiograph (1)?
2. What further investigations are required?

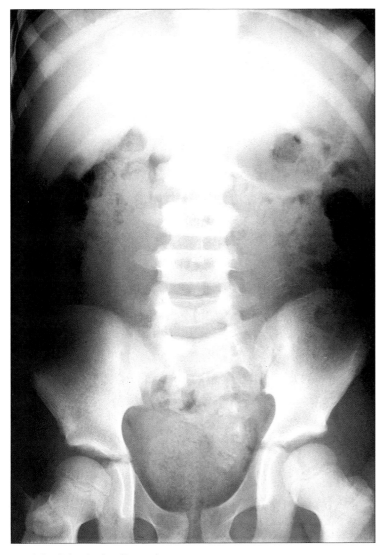

1 Plain abdominal radiograph.

Case 1

3. What abnormalities are seen in **2–6**?
4. What further investigations are indicated?
5. What abnormalities are shown in **7** and **8**?
6. How should this condition be treated?

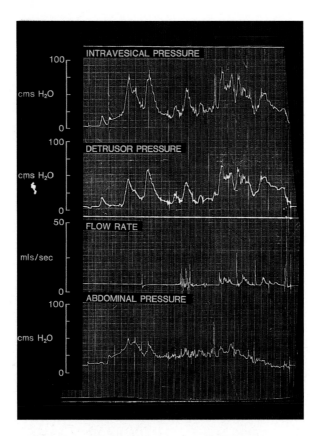

2 Urodynamic pressure trace during filling and voiding.

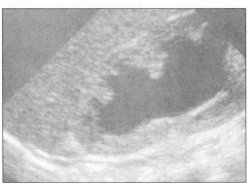

3 Ultrasound scan of right kidney.

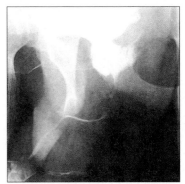

4 Video appearance of bladder and urethra during the voiding phase of the video-urodynamic study.

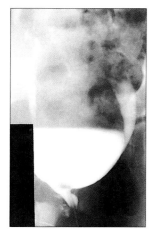

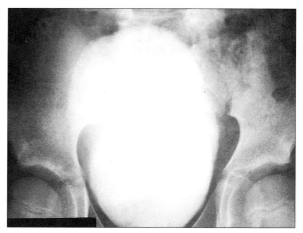

5 Another video appearance of bladder and urethra during the voiding phase of the video-urodynamic study.

6 Bladder after micturition.

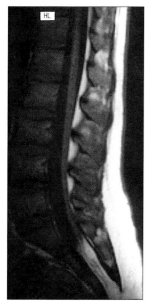

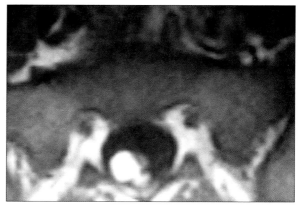

8 Transverse view of MRI of sacral spinal cord.

7 Lateral view of magnetic resonance image (MRI) of sacral spinal cord.

Case 1

1. Partial sacral agenesis with chronic constipation.
2. Renal ultrasound and video-urodynamic studies.
3. **2** shows high-pressure, unstable detrusor contractions during bladder filling, followed by generation of high-pressure detrusor contractions during attempts to void. Urine flow is in small, interrupted spurts of low amplitude. This pattern is typical of detrusor-sphincter dyssynergia, which describes a lack of co-ordination between detrusor and distal urethral sphincter activity, so that the urethra fails to relax during bladder emptying. Bladder emptying is usually incomplete, and urinary tract infections are common. **3** shows right hydronephrosis (the appearance of the left kidney was similar).**4** shows dilatation of the prostatic urethra with narrowing of the membranous urethra during voiding, suggesting failure of the normal reflex relaxation of the distal urethral sphincter. **5** shows vesico-ureteric reflux occurring during voiding as a consequence of high detrusor pressures. **6** shows large post-micturition residue.

   The presence of detrusor-sphincter dyssynergia suggests an underlying spinal cord lesion. The detrusor and distal urethral sphincter are innervated separately from sacral segments S2–4, and co-ordination of their activities is controlled at the level of the pons via long spinal tracts. Supra-sacral spinal cord lesions can interrupt the neural connections between the pons and the sacral micturition centre, resulting in loss of co-ordination of the micturition reflex.
4. As there is a strong suspicion of spinal cord pathology, detailed anatomical imaging of the spinal cord is necessary. The investigation of choice is MRI, but if this facility is not available, myelography may be considered. **9** and **10** show a similar abnormality in another child, diagnosed in an institution where MRI was not available. A filling defect suggesting a sacral lipoma is clearly seen, and again the spinal cord is tethered to the sacrum.

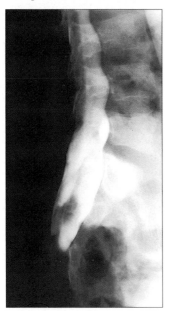 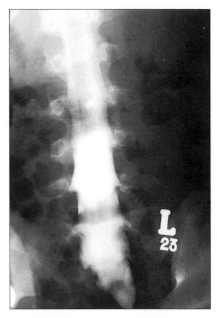

9 Lateral view of myelogram.   **10** Posterior-anterior view of myelogram.

5. A large sacral lipoma communicating with subcutaneous fat and causing spinal cord tethering (**7** and **8**). The spinal cord usually ascends to the adult position level of L1 by the age of two years. In this case, the cord is tethered to the sacrum by the lipoma, preventing normal ascent. As somatic growth occurs, further stretching of the spinal cord and nerve roots can result in progressive neurological deterioration, affecting bladder and bowel function and eventually the lower limbs.

6. Consultation with a neurosurgeon is essential, as restoration of normal bladder control has been reported after successful excision of sacral lipomas. However, surgery is technically demanding, as sacral lipomas tend to be intimately attached to spinal nerve roots, and complete excision without causing further neurological damage may be impossible. In the absence of progressive neuropathy, many neurosurgeons are reluctant to operate.

Conservative management of the bladder pathology consists of administration of anticholinergic medication to reduce detrusor instability and increase functional bladder capacity, combined with intermittent self-catheterisation to empty the bladder regularly and prevent infection.

Case 2
Renal Trauma

A 30-year-old lady fell from a first-floor balcony during a party. She sustained extensive bruising over the back (**1**), and her abdomen was tender and distended, although there was no injury to the bones. She had frank haematuria. There was no clinical evidence of shock, and the serum amylase was within normal limits.

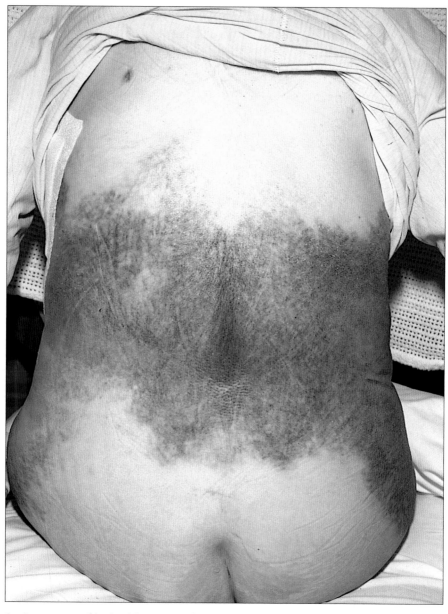

1 Appearance of back with extensive bruising.

QUESTIONS
1. What is the initial radiological investigation of choice?
2. What do the computed tomography (CT) scans show (**2** and **3**)?
3. What is the appropriate initial management?
4. What is the appropriate long-term management?

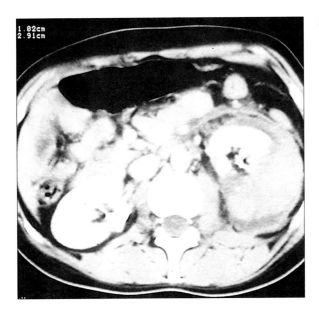

2 Abdominal CT after intravenous contrast medium.

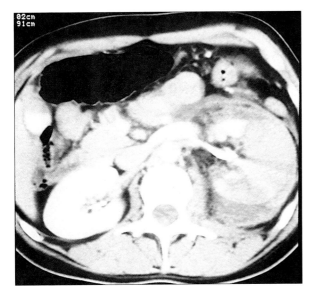

3 Abdominal CT after intravenous contrast medium.

Case 2

ANSWERS

1. An abdominal CT scan with intravenous contrast medium.
2. A normal right kidney and functioning left kidney: a large perinephric haematoma (**2**) and intact renal pedicle (**3**).
3. There is no indication for immediate surgery, provided the patient remains haemodynamically stable. This patient was observed carefully for four days in hospital, during which time her pulse, blood pressure and urine output remained stable and her serum haemoglobin did not fall. By the time of discharge, her abdominal distension had settled, and she had a trace of microscopic haematuria.
4. A CT scan should be repeated several weeks later to check that the haematoma is resolving and to exclude primary renal pathology, which may have been missed by the original study. Kidneys with tumours or congenital anomalies such as pelvi-ureteric junction obstruction are more prone to bleed after trauma than normal kidneys. The patient should also have yearly blood pressure monitoring for life, as perinephric haematomas may cause hypertension in the long term.

Case 3
Right-sided Varicocele

A 25-year-old man presented to his doctor with right-sided scrotal pain. On examination, no abnormalities were found, and an ultrasound scan of the scrotum also showed no abnormalities. Two months later he returned with a complaint of persistent pain, and was found to have a varicocele. He had no other symptoms, and there was no evidence of haematuria on urinalysis. At this stage, the general practitioner arranged for an ultrasound scan of the kidneys, as seen below (1). A CT scan (2) and MRI (3) were also performed.

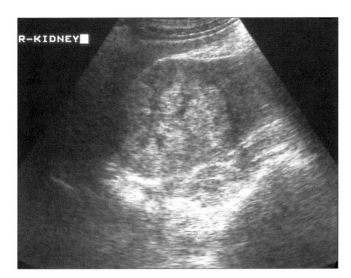

1 Ultrasound scan of right kidney.

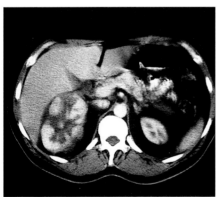

2 CT of abdomen.

3 MRI of abdomen.

QUESTIONS
1. What does the ultrasound show (1)?
2. What is the differential diagnosis?
3. Are any further investigations appropriate prior to surgery?
4. What do the CT and MRI scans show (2 and 3)?
5. Does the imaging information change the surgical management?

Case 3

ANSWERS

1. A solid mass in the upper pole of the right kidney (**4**).

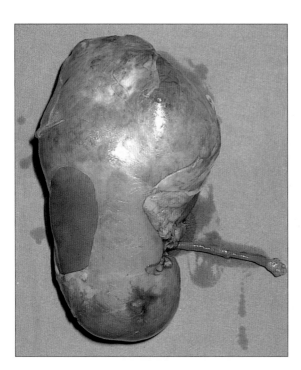

4 Gross appearance of excised right kidney.

2. This is almost certainly a tumour, and renal-cell carcinoma is the most likely diagnosis, although benign tumours should be considered. Varicoceles are more common on the left side in association with renal tumours, and usually suggest renal vein involvement with tumour thrombus causing obstruction to the drainage of the gonadal vein into the renal vein. On the right side, the gonadal vein drains directly into the inferior vena cava, and the presence of a varicocele in association with a tumour is suggestive of a large tumour pressing directly on the gonadal vein.

3. As radical nephrectomy is the treatment of choice for large tumours, further imaging is usually unnecessary. However, CT and MRI imaging may both be helpful in deciding whether the lesion is benign or malignant, and have limited value in the pre-operative assessment of lymph node metastases, although the presence of enlarged lymph nodes does not necessarily imply metastatic involvement. The surgical approach is greatly influenced by the presence of a tumour thrombus in the inferior vena cava, and if this is suspected, the extent of involvement may be more clearly shown by inferior vena cavography. CT-guided biopsy may be useful in certain circumstances, such as: for small tumours when conservative renal surgery may be considered; to make the diagnosis if chemotherapy rather than surgery is to be the primary treatment (e.g. for lymphoma); to confirm the diagnosis if the lesion is considered to be inoperable; or if the patient is unfit for surgery.

4. Both show a large upper pole tumour with the cartwheel appearance typical of an oncocytoma (**5, 6**).

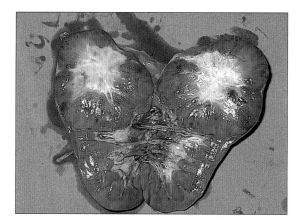

5 Bisected right kidney showing upper pole tumour with cartwheel appearance corresponding to CT and MRI findings.

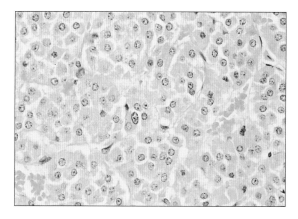

6 Histopathology of oncocytoma showing oncocytes with no evidence of capsular invasion.

5. Although oncocytomas are considered to be benign tumours, they are rare, so the prognosis is not as well documented as for renal-cell carcinomas. Large oncocytomas may have metastatic potential and therefore, in this case, the correct management is right radical nephrectomy, despite information from the CT and MRI scans. There is some evidence that small oncocytomas behave in a benign fashion, so the suspicion of oncocytoma generated by pre-operative imaging may influence the decision in favour of conservative surgery.

Case 4
A Man with Incontinence and Parkinson's Disease

A 60-year-old gentleman with moderate Parkinson's disease presented with a two-year history of frequency, urgency, urge incontinence and a worsening urinary stream. His parkinsonian symptoms were well controlled on madopar and he was able to walk unaided. He had no symptoms of postural hypotension, and no other evidence of autonomic neuropathy. On examination his bladder was not palpable, and his prostate was moderately enlarged and clinically benign. His serum prostate-specific antigen (PSA) was 1.2 µg/l, and his serum creatinine and electrolytes were within normal limits. Urinary tract ultrasound showed no evidence of hydronephrosis, and he had a small-capacity bladder which emptied completely.

QUESTIONS
1. What is the cause of the bladder symptoms?
2. What investigations can be done to differentiate between prostatic obstruction and detrusor hyperreflexia?
3. What information can be derived from these investigations (**1–3**)?
4. How should this patient be managed?

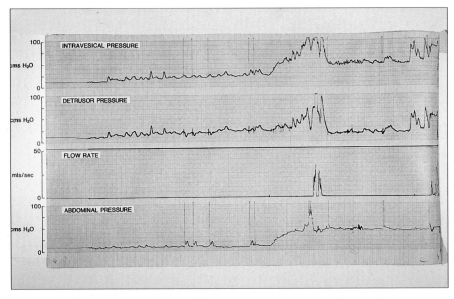

1 Urodynamic pressure trace during filling. Bladder capacity was 150 ml, with unstable contractions of up to 100 cm H_2O during filling.

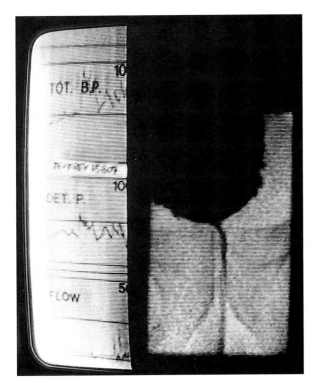

2 Video image of bladder and prostatic urethra during the voiding phase of the urodynamic study. Voiding occurred involuntarily as a result of an unstable contraction, and the bladder emptied completely with a maximum flow rate of 6 ml/sec.

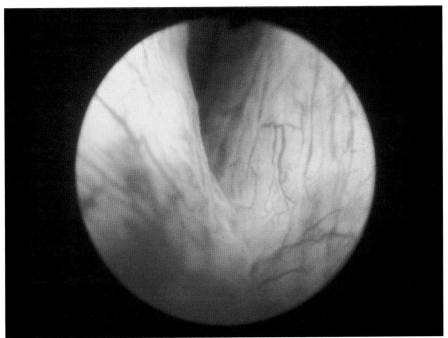

3 Prostatic urethra seen at cysto-urethroscopy.

Case 4

ANSWERS

1. In idiopathic Parkinson's disease with no evidence of dysautonomia, the innervation of the distal urethral sphincter is likely to be intact, so sphincteric incontinence is unlikely. The cause of the bladder symptoms is most likely to be detrusor hyperreflexia or detrusor instability secondary to prostatic obstruction.
2. Video-urodynamic studies and cysto-urethroscopy.
3. The bladder is undoubtedly of low capacity, and detrusor instability or detrusor hyperreflexia is present. Although voiding occurred at a high pressure with a low flow-rate (1), this is not in itself diagnostic of bladder outflow obstruction, as the voiding was involuntary as a result of an unstable detrusor contraction. The voided volume was only 150 ml, so the low flow-rate may not be a reliable recording. The video image (2) shows attenuation of the prostatic urethra, but as the voided volume was small, again this is difficult to interpret.

   The urethroscopic image (3) shows no evidence of middle-lobe enlargement, and the lateral lobes do not appear to be particularly occlusive.
4. It is notoriously difficult to decide whether or not prostatectomy is indicated in men with co-existing neurological conditions and detrusor hyperreflexia. Although detrusor instability secondary to prostatic obstruction would be expected to improve in the majority of cases after prostatectomy, detrusor hyperreflexia can be made worse, and as this patient is suffering from urgency and urge incontinence, the morbidity associated with prostatectomy is probably unjustified in the first instance. A trial of anticholinergic medication, such as oxybutynin, is worthwhile, but there is a risk of precipitating acute urinary retention.

   Alternatives to prostatectomy should be considered, and drug treatment with alpha blockers or 5-alpha reductase inhibitors would be appropriate initial therapy, since neither interact with madopar. A favourable symptomatic response to medical treatment would suggest that prostatic obstruction is the main cause for the symptoms, and would indicate that subsequent prostatectomy is likely to be successful. On the other hand, if medical therapy is more acceptable to the patient, there is no reason why this should not be continued on a permanent basis, provided long-term follow-up is undertaken to monitor possible upper tract deterioration or the development of prostate cancer.

   Procedures such as thermotherapy, laser therapy and prostatic stenting may also be considered, but again, long-term follow-up is essential.

Case 5
A Hazard of Sleeping

A 38-year-old man presented to the emergency department at 0400 hours having developed severe penile pain after rolling over in bed. On examination there was obvious bruising of the penis (**1**).

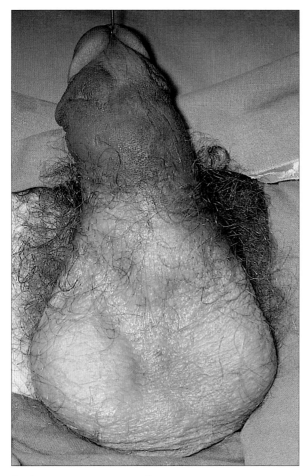

1 Appearance at presentation.

QUESTIONS
1. What is the suspected diagnosis?
2. What is the best immediate management?
3. What long-term complications may result, and how should they be treated?

Case 5

ANSWERS

1. Fractured penis, i.e. rupture of the tunica albuginea of the corpus cavernosum. This injury occurs when the erect penis if forcibly bent, usually during sexual intercourse. There is often a loud cracking noise followed by immediate detumescence and bruising. Associated urethral injury can occur.

2. Diagnosis is usually on the history and clinical findings alone, and usually no special investigations are required. If urethral injury is suspected, a urethrogram is indicated.

   The best treatment is immediate surgical evacuation of the haematoma and repair of the tear in the tunica albuginea (**2–4**). This can usually be performed via a subcoronal incision using absorbable sutures such as 3/0 vicryl or polydioxanone (PDS). Any urethral injury can be repaired at the same time. Conservative management of the injury is not recommended, due to the high incidence of late complications.

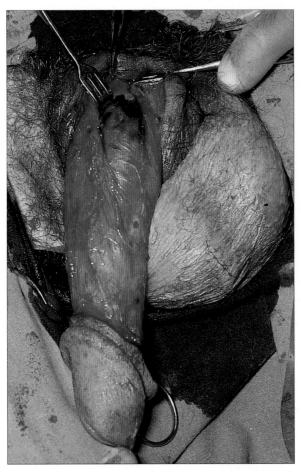

2 Operative appearance showing tear in tunica albuginea and its repair.

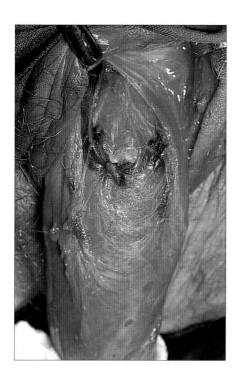

3 Operative appearance showing tear in tunica albuginea and its repair.

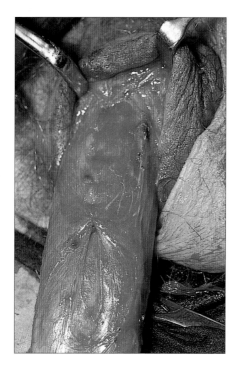

4 Operative appearance showing tear in tunica albuginea and its repair.

Case 5

3. The commonest long-term complications after a fractured penis are either failure of, or deformity, on erection, a condition similar to Peyronie's disease (**5**). Both these problems arise due to corporal fibrosis. If deformity is the main problem, it may be corrected by a Nesbit operation or modifications thereof, but if there is concomitant erectile failure, the only suitable option may be implantation of a semi-rigid or inflatable penile prosthesis.

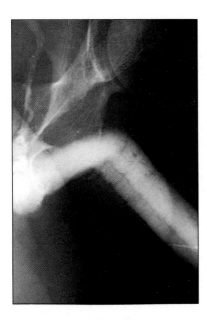

5 Corpus cavernosogram demonstrates extreme angulation of shaft due to Peyronie plaque. (Reprinted from Lloyd–Davies, W. Parkhouse, H., Gow, J. and Davies, D., *Color Atlas of Urology, Second Edition*, London, Wolfe Publishing, 1994.)

Case 6
A Neonate with Vesico-ureteric Reflux

A male fetus was found to have bilateral hydronephrosis at 16 weeks' gestation; serial scans showed normal bladder emptying with persistent bilateral hydronephrosis, but no evidence of oligohydramnios. No chromosomal abnormalities were detected on amniocentesis.

The baby was delivered spontaneously at full term and had a good Apgar score. Serum creatinine concentration was within normal limits. An ultrasound scan on the first day of life (1) showed bilateral hydro-ureteronephrosis with no evidence of bladder wall thickening.

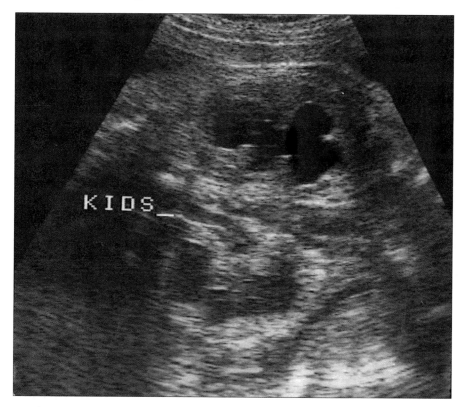

1 Ultrasound scan on the first day of life.

QUESTIONS
1. What further radiological investigations should be done as soon as possible after birth (see **2** and **3**, overleaf)?
2. What do these investigations show?
3. How should this condition be managed initially?
4. At the age of six months, the baby developed a urinary tract infection with *Escherichia coli* despite regular antibiotic prophylaxis. How should this situation be managed?
5. What does the isotope scan show (see **4**, overleaf)?
6. How does this finding alter management?
7. What is the long-term management?

Case 6

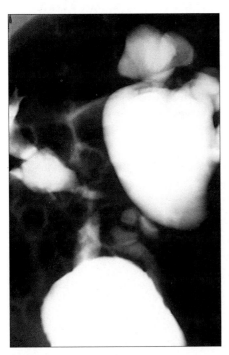

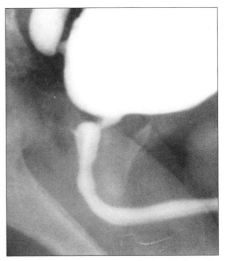

3 Voiding phase of micturating cysto-urethrogram (with antibiotic cover) on first day of life.

2 Filling phase of micturating cysto-urethrogram (with antibiotic prophylaxis) on first day of life.

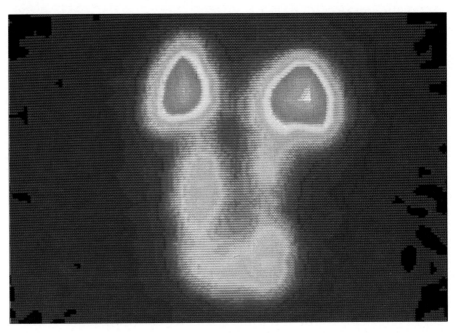

4 Isotope cystogram showing persistent bilateral reflux.

ANSWERS

1. Micturating cysto-urethrogram (MCUG) (**2** and **3**).
2. Micturating cysto-urethrogram shows bilateral vesico-ureteric reflux (**2**) with no evidence of urethral obstruction (**3**).
3. It is of vital importance to prevent urinary tract infection, as infection in the presence of vesico-ureteric reflux may lead to acute pyelonephritis, which can ultimately cause permanent renal scarring. Antibiotic prophylaxis should be started immediately; the most commonly used antibiotic is trimethoprim (2 mg/kg/day). Regular urine testing for infection should be carried out, and if the baby develops a febrile illness, urinary tract infection should be excluded as a matter of urgency.

   It is also important to establish baseline functional imaging of the kidneys prior to the occurrence of urinary tract infection in order to be able to detect possible scars in the future. The baseline imaging may already show abnormalities due to renal dysplasia, which commonly accompanies vesico-ureteric reflux. The most commonly used investigation for functional renal parenchymal imaging is isotope scintigraphy using technetium dimerocaptosuccinic acid (Tc^{99m}DMSA), which provides a static image of functioning renal tubules and differential renal function. This isotope is not handled well by the neonatal kidney, and imaging should be deferred until the age of 1 month (**5**). It is also important to exclude obstruction in the upper tracts, as conditions such as pelvi-ureteric junction obstruction may co-exist with vesico-ureteric reflux. Renography with Tc^{99m}MAG 3 may help to exclude obstruction, although the investigation can be equivocal in the first few months of life.
4. The baby should be treated with an intravenous antibiotic according to the sensitivity of the organism. Tc^{99m}DMSA scintigraphy should be repeated at least three weeks after the acute infection, in order to assess whether any permanent renal scarring has occurred. Imaging during acute infection may lead to false-positive results.

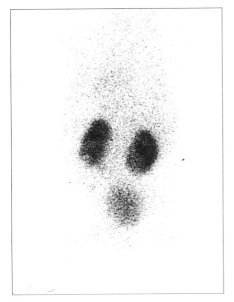

5 Normal Tc^{99m}DMSA scan at one month.

Case 6

5. Bilateral photon deficient areas (**6**). As the previous scan was normal, this new finding is compatible with renal scarring following acute infection.
6. As a breakthrough infection has already occurred on prophylactic antibiotic medication, continuation of conservative treatment is unlikely to prevent further infection, and therefore consideration should now be given to anti-reflux surgery. As vesico-ureteric reflux will resolve spontaneously in most cases, the indications for open surgery are controversial. Although ureteric reimplantation is technically possible at the age of six months, and there is a greater than 90% chance of curing the reflux, there is a small risk of damage to the vas deferens or seminal vesicles which may contribute to subfertility in adult life.

   As an alternative to open surgery, subtrigonal injection of Polytef ©, collagen or macroplastique © into the ureteric orifices via an infant cysto-urethroscope is a useful technique, which is a relatively complication-free method of producing temporary resolution of reflux in the hope that spontaneous resolution will ultimately occur.

   Prior to surgery, it is necessary to confirm the persistence of reflux, and this can be done with an isotope cystogram (**4**), which carries less radiation risk than a contrast micturating cystogram.
7. After resolution of reflux, it is necessary to monitor renal function and blood pressure in the long term, as complications from renal scarring may occur at any time in the future.

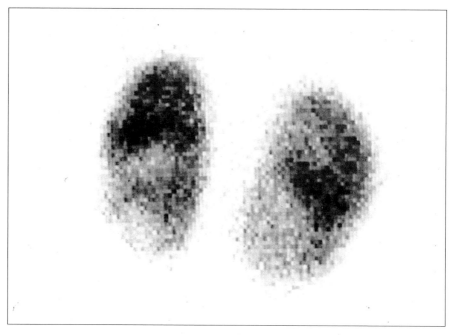

6 Tc^{99m}DMSA scan three weeks after acute urinary tract infection.

Case 7
Hypertension

A 55-year-old woman presented to her general practitioner with headaches, and was found to have a blood pressure of 180/120 mmHg. **1** and **2** show her skin condition on presentation.

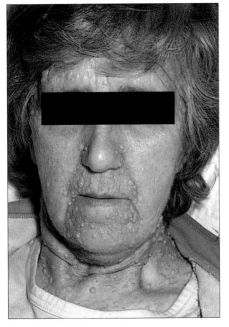

1 Patient's face.

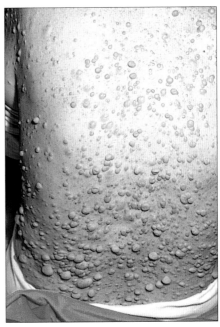

2 Patient's back.

QUESTIONS
1. What is the spot diagnosis (**1** and **2**)?
2. What specific causes of hypertension are associated with this condition?
3. What investigations should be done?
4. What abnormality is seen in **3**?
5. What is the diagnosis and treatment?

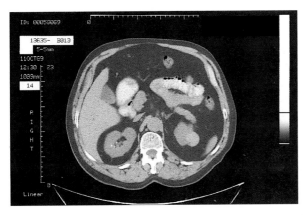

3 Abdominal CT.

Case 7

ANSWERS

1. Neurofibromatosis (**1** and **2**).
2. Renovascular disease and pheochromocytoma.
3. 24-hour urine collection for measurement of unconjugated catecholamines and vanillylmandelic acid (VMA); intravenous digital subtraction angiography of the aorta and renal arteries; and abdominal CT (**3**).

   In this case, the urinary catecholamines were raised, and digital vascular imaging showed no abnormalities.
4. Left-sided adrenal tumour (**3**).
5. The tumour is in undoubtedly in the adrenal gland in the CT scan, and the abnormal urinary catecholamines differentiate a phaeochromocytoma from other types of adrenal tumour. Treatment is surgical. Prior to surgery, the blood pressure should be well controlled with alpha blockers. Thoracic tumours should be excluded by CT.

   The tumour should be explored via a transabdominal or thoraco-abdominal incision, so that a careful laparotomy can be performed in order to exclude further extra-adrenal tumours, which may have been missed on pre-operative imaging.

   Post-operatively, urinary catecholamine levels should ultimately return to normal. Failure to do so is indicative of further undiagnosed tumours or malignancy (although most phaeochromocytomas are benign).

   4 shows the excised left adrenal gland with left kidney. **5** shows the tumour bisected. Note the characteristic colour of the phaeochromocytoma, in contrast to the pallor of a Conn's tumour (**6**). **7** shows the histopathological characteristics of a phaeochromocytoma.

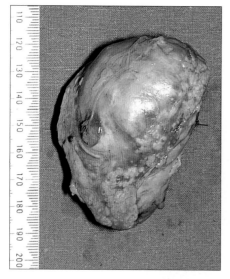 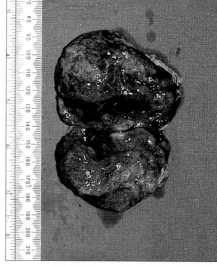

4 Excised left adrenal gland and kidney.   **5** Tumour bisected.

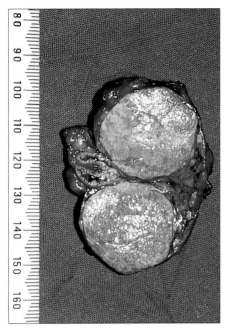

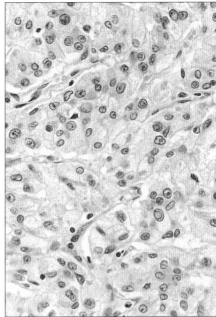

6 Conn's tumour bisected.

7 Phaeochromocytoma on microscopy.

Case 8
Gynaecomastia

A 26-year-old man presented to his GP with mild bilateral gynaecomastia (1). He was reassured that this was normal, and he had no investigations or treatment. Three years later he presented to his local accident and emergency department with acute abdominal pain, and an emergency laparotomy was carried out. A large, retroperitoneal mass was found which was biopsied, and the abdomen was closed. The histology showed a malignant teratoma with some undifferentiated elements.

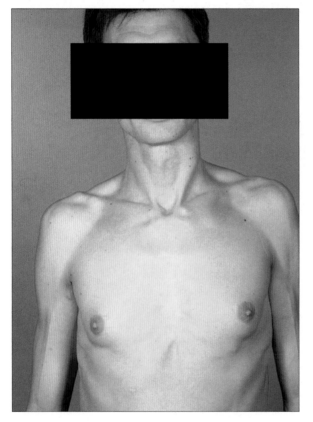

1 Patient's chest showing bilateral gynaecomastia.

QUESTIONS
1. What further investigations should be done?
2. What do the radiological investigations show (2–4)?
3. What further investigations should be done on the basis of these findings?
4. What do these show, and what treatment is appropriate?
5. Following chemotherapy, the chest metastases and brain metastases regressed, and the serum human chorionic gonadotrophin (HCG) dropped to 1,000 IU/l. What does the post-treatment abdominal CT show (5)?
6. What is the most appropriate way to manage this situation?

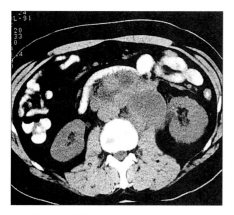

2 CT scan of abdomen.

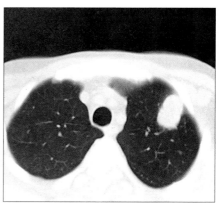

3 CT scan of chest.

4 CT scan of chest.

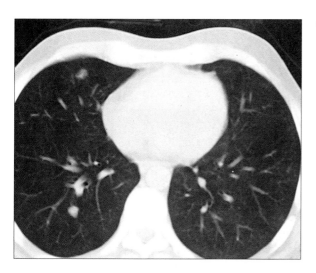

5 Post-treatment abdominal CT scan.

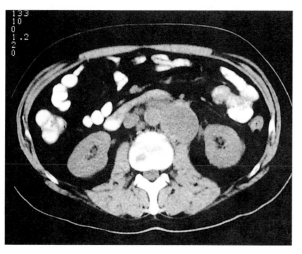

Case 8

ANSWERS

1. Examination and ultrasound scan of testes revealed no abnormalities. Serum alphafetoprotein (AFP) was normal, but serum HCG was 500,000 IU/l. The CT scans of the abdomen and chest are shown (2–4).
2. The abdominal CT (2) shows bulky para-aortic lymphadenopathy with lateral displacement of left kidney but no hydronephrosis. The chest CT scan shows a large metastasis in the left lung (3) and multiple metastases in right lung (4).
3. An MRI scan of the brain, as there is a 20% chance of asymptomatic brain metastases in stage IV disease (6, 7).
4. Left-sided parietal metastasis (6) and right-sided occipital metastasis (7). Treatment consists of systemic chemotherapy with a platinum-based regimen in combination with etoposide, and with additional intrathecal chemotherapy.
5. The post-chemotherapy abdominal CT (5) shows residual para-aortic disease, but this has reduced in size, showing a favourable response to chemotherapy.
6. Retroperitoneal lymph node dissection to remove all residual abdominal tumour should be performed. Post-operatively, further treatment depends on the histology of the excised tissue and the tumour marker response.

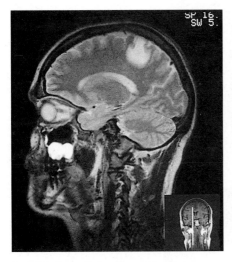

6 MRI of saggital section of brain.

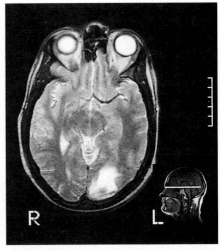

7 MRI of coronal section of brain.

Case 9
Haematuria?

A man aged 69, having noticed blood stains on his underpants for about one year, was referred by his general practitioner to a haematuria clinic. No clinical examination had been performed prior to his attendance. On examination, there was an obvious lesion of his penis (**1**).

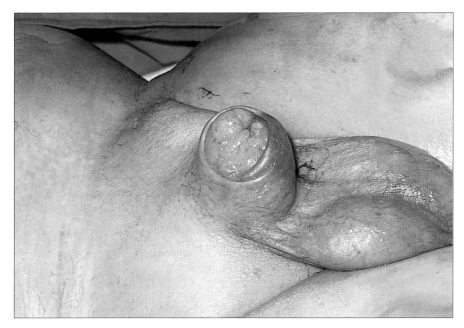

1 Appearance at presentation.

QUESTIONS
1 What abnormalities are shown?
2. What is the differential diagnosis?
3. What factors predispose to this condition?
4. What treatment options exist?

Case 9

1. There is a squamous carcinoma of the penis. There is also a left inguinal swelling, suggesting the possibility of secondary lymphadenopathy.
2. Carcinoma of the penis should be distinguished from genital warts (condyloma accuminatum), in particular the giant condyloma known as the Buschke–Löwenstein tumour (2). This is an exophytic lesion which grows slowly, and may progressively destroy the penis. Cases of overtly malignant change in such a tumour are exceedingly rare, and it rarely metastasises. Histologically, the tumour is well differentiated and shows no signs of vascular or lymphatic invasion. If the diagnosis is thus confirmed, the tumour can be treated by conservative excision with good results.

   Other rare primary tumours occurring in the penis include basal-cell carcinomas, melanomas, lymphomas and sarcomas. Secondary penile tumours are also rare, and usually represent spread from the prostate or bladder.
3. Carcinoma of the penis always occurs in uncircumcised men. It is common in China, India and the Far East, and also in uncircumcised African tribes. There have been reports of an increased incidence of cervical carcinomas in partners of men with carcinoma of the penis, possibly linking it with herpes virus infection. In the West it is usually diagnosed in the seventh or eighth decades of life.

   Pre-malignant conditions include leucoplakia and erythroplasia of Queyrat or Bowen's disease (3 and 4), both of which are essentially *in situ* penile carcinomas. These latter conditions present as velvety, well-circumscribed lesions, with cells showing hyperchromatic nuclei with many mitotic figures (5) whose appearances contrast with those of a carcinoma (6). There have also been occasional reports of malignant change in patients with balanitis xerotica obliterans.

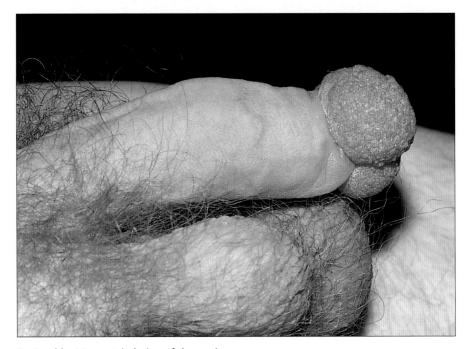

2 Buschke-Löwenstein lesion of the penis.

Case 9

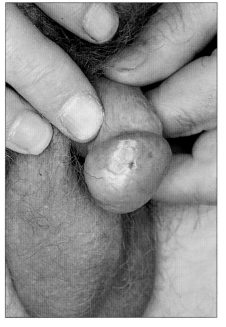

3 Erythroplasia of Queyrat.

4 Microscopic appearance of erythroplasia of Queyrat. (low power)

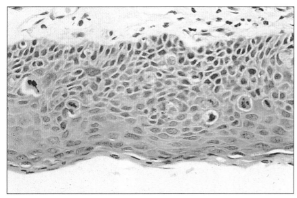

5 Microscopic appearance of erythroplasia of Queyrat (high power).

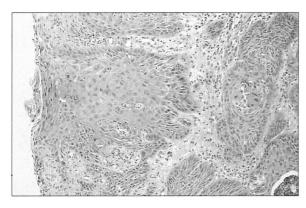

6 Microscopic appearance of squamous carcinoma of the penis.

4. Initial treatment of squamous carcinomas is either surgical or by using radiotherapy. Circumcision alone leaves a high risk of local recurrence. Therefore, for distal lesions, partial amputation of the penis is recommended (**7, 8**) whilst for more proximal lesions a radical amputation with or without bilateral orchiectomy may be required. Radiotherapy may be preferred in younger patients or those who wish to remain sexually active, but it is best suited to small distal tumours. Although penile anatomy may be preserved, an adequate dose of irradiation may result in significant side-effects such as pain, oedema and urethral stricture or fistula.

The question of unilateral or bilateral block dissection of the inguinal nodes remains controversial. It should only be undertaken if nodes persist after eradication of infection, and its likely survival benefits have to be weighed against its proven morbidity.

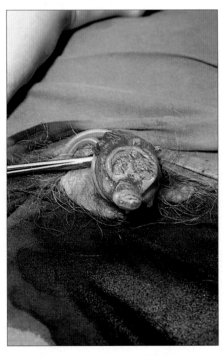

7 Partial amputation of the penis.

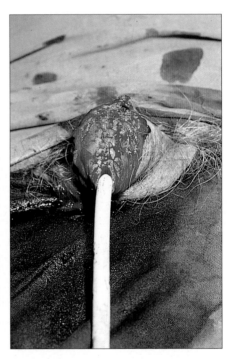

8 Partial amputation of the penis.

Case 10
Spontaneous Fractures

A 60-year-old lady who sustained an extra-capsular fracture of the right hip had no history of trauma. The fracture was reduced and fixed, and a specimen of bone from the fracture site was sent for histological examination. There was no evidence of tumour or osteoporosis on histological examination. A hip radiograph one month later (**1**) showed good evidence of healing.

Two months later, she sustained a second spontaneous fracture at the same site (**2**). After complaining of back pain with no previous history of trauma, a spontaneous wedge fracture of L3 vertebra was discovered. A bone scan, thyroid scan, mammography and bone densimetry were all normal. Serum calcium concentration (corrected) was normal, but serum parathyroid hormone (PTH) was grossly elevated.

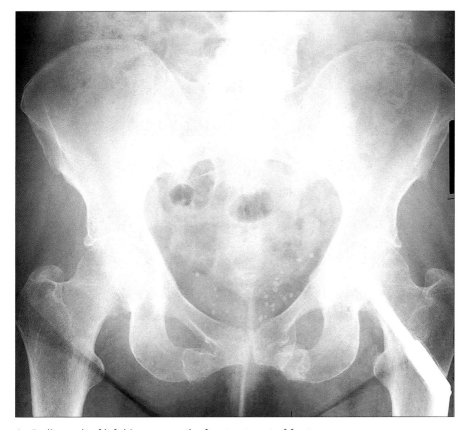

1 Radiograph of left hip one month after treatment of fracture.

Case 10

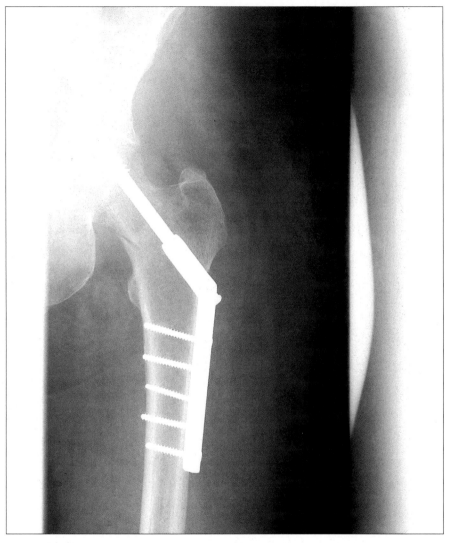

2 Radiograph of left hip three months after treatment of fracture, showing re-fracture.

QUESTIONS
1. What is the most likely diagnosis?
2. What further investigations are indicated?
3. What does the 2-methoxy isobutyl isonitrile (MIBI) scan (**3**) show?
4. What is the correct management?

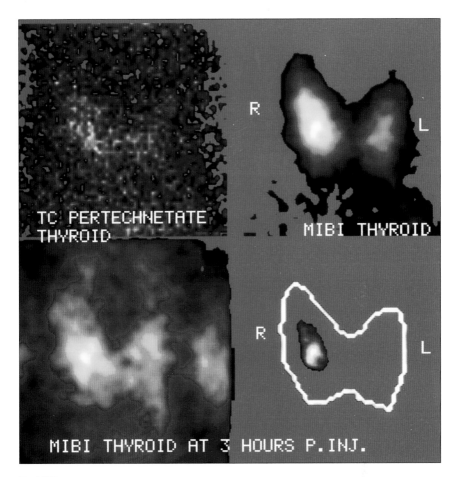

3 MIBI scan.

ANSWERS

1. In view of the elevated PTH, despite the normal calcium, primary hyper-parathyroidism is the most likely diagnosis.
2. The serum calcium should be repeated on several occasions until hypercalcaemia is detected. If hypercalcaemia is diagnosed in conjunction with a raised PTH, then surgical exploration of the parathyroid glands is required. The steroid suppression test, although commonly used, has a low sensitivity and specificity for parathyroid disease. Isotope scanning of the parathyroid glands may be useful for locating ectopic tissue, but is not essential prior to surgery.
3. Abnormal activity in the right upper parathyroid.
4. Exploration of the neck. Although abnormal activity was only shown in the right upper parathyroid, it is important to explore all four parathyroid glands and to remove any obvious adenomatous tissue. If there is any suspicion of parathyroid hyperplasia, it may be necessary to biopsy all four glands for frozen section and histological analysis.

Bilateral Ureteric Obstruction (1)

A 64-year-old painter presented with a two-month history of intermittent macroscopic haematuria. There were no other urological symptoms, and his health was previously good. He smoked 20 cigarettes a day, took no drugs and had never travelled abroad. There were no abnormal findings on physical examination.

A mid-stream urine sample showed > 50 red blood cells (RBC)/hpf without growth. Urine cytology was negative. His haemoglobin, serum creatinine and electrolytes were all normal.

QUESTIONS

1. Describe the abnormal findings of the intravenous urogram (IVU) (**1**). What is the differential diagnosis?
2. What other investigations would you perform?
3. What are the risk factors associated with these abnormalities?
4. What treatment options exist?
5. What further treatment should be considered?

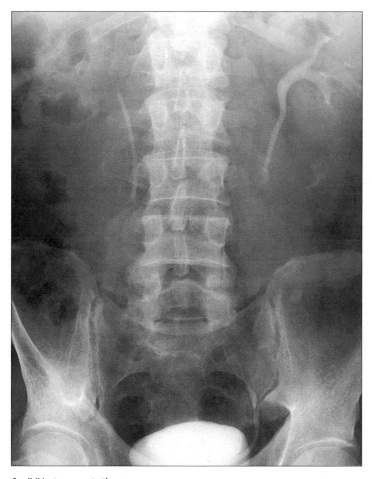

1 IVU at presentation.

ANSWERS

1. The IVU shows filling defects in both ureters, most probably due to transitional-cell tumours. The differential diagnosis includes radiolucent stones and ureteritis cystica.

2. Cystoscopy is mandatory, as approximately 50% of patients with upper urinary tract tumours have associated lesions in their bladders. Retrograde ureterography should be performed (2), and at the same time urine can be taken from each ureter and sent for cytology. In this case, cytology was negative, as the tumours were of low grade. Antegrade pyelography is usually contraindicated, as tumour may be seeded along the puncture track. CT scanning may help in assessing the degree of invasiveness and operability of the tumours. If there is real difficulty in establishing the diagnosis, ureteroscopy may be useful. In addition, if there is ureteric obstruction and doubt about the useful function of either kidney, a $Tc^{99m}DMSA$ renogram may be indicated.

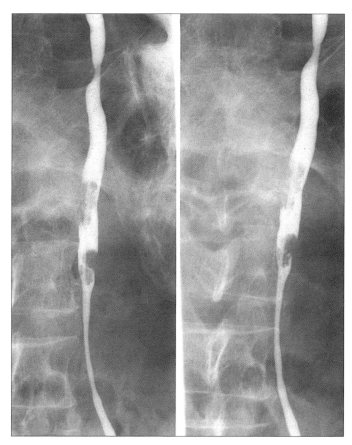

2 Retrograde ureterogram showing ureteric tumour.

In this case, the left ureterogram shows two fairly substantial left ureteric tumours. The right ureterogram showed only a small tumour on that side.

Case 11

3. Ureteric tumors are rare before the age of 40, and are commoner in men. They are associated with smoking and analgesic abuse, and possibly with heavy coffee-drinking. They are common in Balkan countries in association with a nephropathy. Various occupations are associated with an increased risk of forming urothelial tumours—these include car and leather workers, and those exposed to organic chemicals. Painters, as in this case, are also at increased risk.

4. For unilateral upper tract tumours, the standard treatment is a radical nephroureterectomy. This is acceptable as the risk of developing a contralateral upper tract tumour is only 2–4%. Where the tumours are bilateral or in solitary kidneys, it is appropriate to consider more conservative surgery. In this case, the patient underwent a right nephroureterectomy. The left ureteric tumour was excised by a small ureterotomy, and the ureter repaired over a double pigtail stent (**3**). The patient was then followed up by regular urine cytology and check cystoscopies with annual retrograde ureterograms.

Four years later, he re-presented with a short history of general malaise and oliguria. Routine investigations confirmed him to be in acute renal failure with a serum creatinine of 1024 μmol/l. Haemodialysis was commenced, and further radiological investigations confirmed extensive tumour of the left ureter.

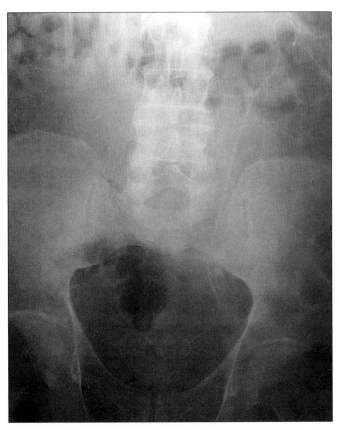

3 Left double pigtail stent in ureter following right nephroureterectomy and local excision of left ureteric tumour.

5. If the tumour remains low-grade and small, a further excision or resection may be possible. If, however, it is more extensive (as was the case here), the patient should undergo a total ureterectomy with replacement of the defect with a bowel segment, commonly ileum (**4**). The only alternative to a bowel interposition is to consider renal auto transplantation. For patients not considered suitable for surgery, there have been reports of successful courses of chemotherapeutic agents (e.g. mitomycin C or bacillus Calmette–Guerin [BCG]) instilled into the bladder (if vesico-ureteric reflux is present) or directly into the ureters.

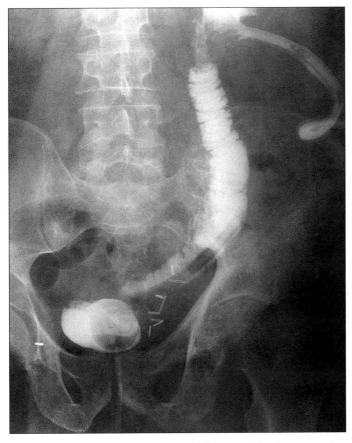

4 Antegrade ureterogram showing ileal interposition between left renal pelvis and bladder following total ureterectomy.

Case 12
Bilateral Ureteric Obstruction (2)

A 64-year-old obese lady presented with a four-week history of backache, weight loss and general malaise. On examination there were no abnormal findings. Her erythrocyte sedimentation rate (ESR) was 81 mm/hr, and serum creatinine was elevated at 161 µmol/l.

QUESTIONS
1. What is shown by the IVU (1) and ultrasound scan (2), and what is the diagnosis?
2. What are the common causes of this condition?
3. How should this condition be managed?

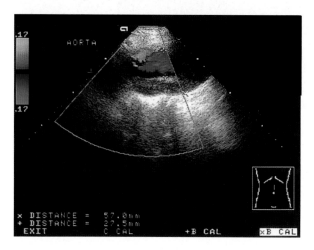

1 IVU at presentation.

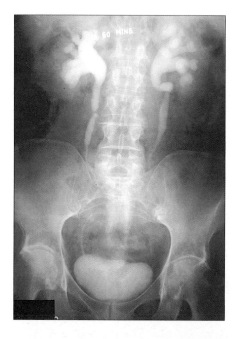

2 Colour-duplex ultrasound showing 5.7-cm aortic aneurysm containing thrombus.

ANSWERS

1. There is a bilateral ureteric obstruction with some medial displacement of the ureters. In conjunction with the raised ESR, the diagnosis is of retroperitoneal fibrosis (RPF). The ultrasound scan shows a large abdominal aortic aneurysm.

2. Over 50% of cases of RPF are idiopathic. There is an association between RPF and aneurysmal disease of the aorta (either inflammatory or otherwise), and it has been suggested that a lipoprotein—ceroid—leaking through the aortic wall may initiate an IgG-mediated reaction, causing fibrosis. Other benign causes include drugs such as methyldopa, methysergide and ergot derivatives, inflammatory bowel disease, infections and fat necrosis. Any retroperitoneal malignancy, but especially lymphomas and metastatic carcinoma, may cause similar extrinsic ureteric compression.

3. Whenever possible, the aetiology of the condition should be established and treatment directed at the cause. In this case, therefore, it would be appropriate to repair the patient's aortic aneurysm. When no aneurysm exists, a CT scan (**3**) is usually performed, and a percutaneous needle biopsy of abnormal tissue may be taken. This is a useful test if malignancy is confirmed, but there is a high false-negative rate with such biopsies. It is therefore sometimes necessary to perform a laparotomy and biopsy to establish diagnosis, and in this case a ureterolysis should be performed. In this procedure, the ureter or ureters are moved laterally and intraperitonealised so that further obstruction cannot occur (**4**). If operative intervention is not indicated, double pigtail stents can be inserted into the renal pelves to prevent obstruction. Oral steroids are also sometimes helpful. Follow-up should consist of long-term monitoring of renal function.

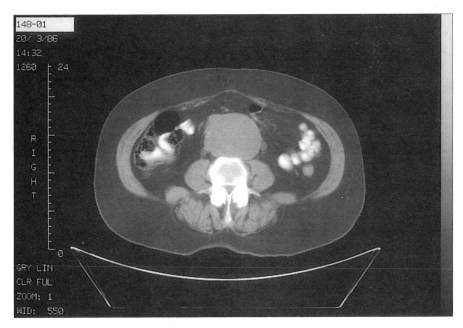

3 CT scan confirming abdominal aortic aneurysm.

Case 12

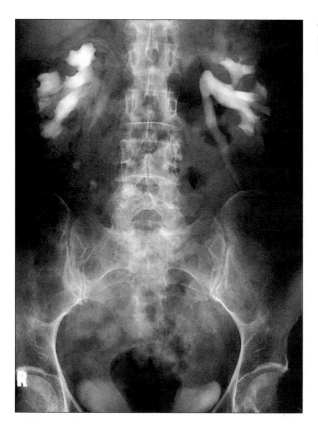

4 IVU after ureterolysis, showing lateral displacement of ureters.

Case 13
Azoospermia

During investigation of a couple's infertility, the 28-year-old man was found to be azoospermic. There was no relevant current or past medical history. Physical examination revealed normal secondary sexual characteristics. Both testes were of normal size, the vasa deferentia were normal, but both epididymes were distended (1). Semen analysis showed complete azoospermia with a semen volume of 0.5 ml, pH 6.0 and absent fructose.

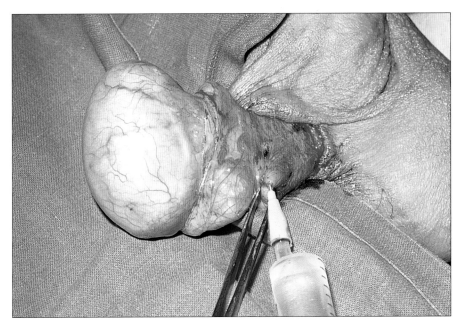

1 Operative slide showing epididymal distension. The cannula is inserted into the distal vas ready for vasography.

QUESTIONS
1. What is the most likely diagnosis?
2. What are the major causes of this problem?
3. What further investigations should be performed?

Case 13

ANSWERS

1. The low volume and pH of the ejaculate, and the absence of fructose, suggest a diagnosis of ejaculatory duct obstruction.
2. Obstruction may be due to congenital causes, such as Mullerian duct cysts, seminal vesicle abnormalities or ejaculatory duct agenesis, trauma, infections such as prostatitis or epididymitis, and rarely, prostatic or seminal vesicle neoplasms.
3. The serum follicle-stimulating hormone (FSH), luteinising hormone (LH) and testosterone should be measured. Elevation of FSH and LH above twice the normal maximum suggests a diagnosis of primary testicular failure, in which case further investigation is unlikely to be of practical use. Transrectal ultrasound and MRI scanning can be used to provide more detailed information as to seminal vesicle anatomy, but were not done in this case.

If the serum hormone levels are normal, a scrotal exploration should be undertaken to perform vasography for seeking the site and nature of an obstruction. Testicular biopsies are performed at the same time to ensure that normal spermatogenesis is occurring. In this case, exploration of the right testis revealed a grossly distended epididymis (**1**), and vasography (**2**) showed obstruction due to a müllerian duct cyst with no contrast entering the bladder. Testicular biopsies were normal (**3**). Cysto-urethroscopy confirmed the presence of the cyst, which was immediately incised. This resulted in the discharge of thick brown fluid and the restoration of a normal sperm count by six weeks postoperatively.

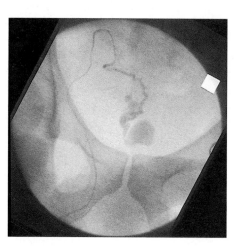

2 Right vasogram showing normal vas deferens and seminal vesicle. Contrast accumulates in the müllerian cyst.

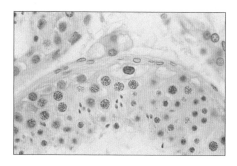

3 Testicular biopsy (× 150) showing stages of normal spermatogenesis with progression from spermatogonia to spermatocytes and spermatids.

Case 14
Backache and Voiding Difficulty

A 57-year-old man presented with a three-month history of low backache, a reduced urinary stream and nocturia × 3. On examination, his bladder was palpable halfway to the umbilicus, and his prostate was enlarged and contained a hard nodule in the right lobe. Serum creatinine was elevated at 316 μmol/l, and prostate-specific antigen (PSA) was elevated at 126 ng/ml. A transrectal ultrasound scan and biopsy of his prostate was performed (**1** and **2**).

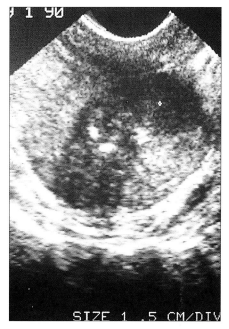

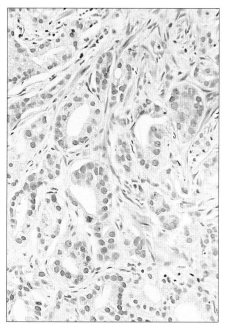

1 Transrectal ultrasound of the prostate. The dot marks a hypo-echoic lesion ready to be biopsied.

2 Microscopic appearance of prostate biopsy.

QUESTIONS
1. What is shown by the scan and biopsy?
2. What immediate treatment is required?
3. What further investigations may be helpful?

Case 14

ANSWERS

1. The scan shows hypo-echoic areas in both lobes of the prostate with some deformity of the capsule. This is in keeping with the likely diagnosis of a prostatic carcinoma which is confirmed histologically.
2. A urinary catheter should be inserted as the patient is in chronic retention with renal failure. Relief of the obstruction may result in a diuresis, necessitating replacement of fluids intravenously. Once renal function is stable, a transurethral prostatectomy can be performed.
3. If renal function fails to improve, an ultrasound of the kidneys should be performed, both to determine cortical size and any evidence of ureteric obstruction. Bone scans are often performed to look for evidence of secondary tumour spread, but it is now clear that they are virtually always normal in patients with PSA levels < 20 mg/ml. In this case, a bone scan was performed (**3**).

3 Bone scan.

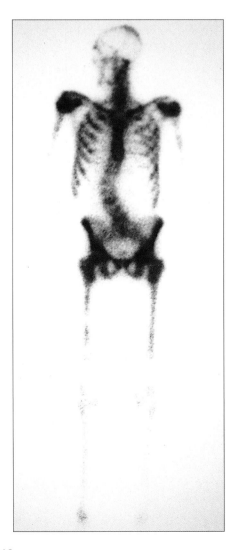

QUESTIONS

4. What is shown by the bone scan (**3**)?
5. What treatment should be undertaken?

ANSWERS

4. The appearances are those of a 'superscan'. Although the symmetrical and diffuse uptake may give the impression of a normal scan, this appearance is due to widespread metastases. As all the isotope is taken up into bone, the kidneys are not visualised.
5. The initial treatment should involve restoring normal bladder emptying by a transurethral prostatectomy. Due to the secondary spread of the tumour, local, possibly curative treatment is not possible. Hormonal manipulation with anti-androgens or luteinising hormone-releasing hormone (LHRH) antagonists can be commenced, and response monitored by serial PSA measurements; a rapid fall to normal values indicates a significantly better prognosis than a lesser response.

PROGRESS

After the above treatment, the patient did well for six months. He then re-presented with a one-week history of severe back pain and difficulty in walking. On examination, there was bilateral lower limb weakness with reduced sensation below the level of T12.

QUESTIONS

6. What is the likely diagnosis?
7. What further action should be taken?

Case 14

ANSWERS

6. Spinal cord compression due to secondary tumour.
7. Intravenous dexamethasone (4 mg t.d.s.) should be started. Myelography or, more recently, an MRI scan can be performed to define the extent of the disease (**4** and **5**). The choice of further treatment lies between radiotherapy and spinal decompression. The latter is probably only helpful if there is a solitary spinal deposit. Treatment must be commenced immediately if there is to be any realistic chance of recovery of lower limb function.

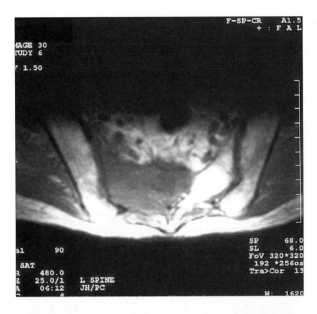

4 MRI scan (transverse view) showing destruction of sacrum by tumour.

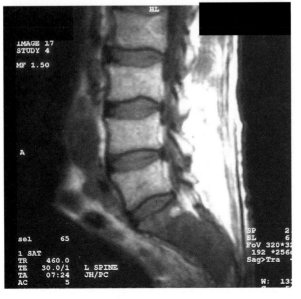

5 MRI scan (sagittal view). In addition to the sacral lesion, there is a small deposit in the L2 vertebra.

Case 15
A Farming Injury

A 30-year-old farmer presented as an emergency case, having fallen off a tractor onto a spiked roller. He had sustained a penetrating perineal injury (1), and there was blood at his external urethral meatus. He was otherwise totally unharmed. A urethrogram was performed (2).

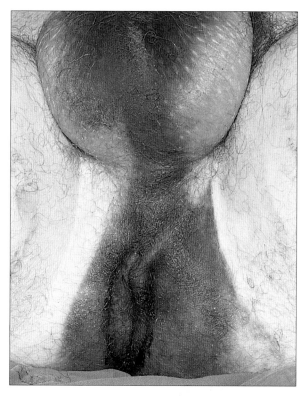

1 Appearance at presentation.

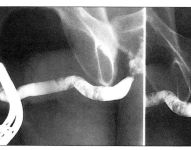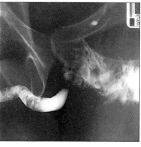

2 Urethrogram at presentation.

QUESTIONS
1. What physical sign is shown in the picture of the original injury (**1**)?
2. What is shown by the urethrogram (**2**)?
3. What is the most appropriate initial management for this patient?
4. How should the patient be managed thereafter?

Case 15

ANSWERS

1. The picture (**1**) shows a butterfly haematoma due to extravasation of blood within the confines of Colles' fascia in the perineum. The scrotal bruising may thus extend onto the anterior abdominal wall.

2. The urethrogram (**2**) (which should be performed with water-soluble contrast) confirms the urethral disruption with leakage of contrast posteriorly and no contrast entering the bladder.

3. A suprapubic catheter should be inserted, if need be, at open cystotomy. Sigmoidoscopy should also be performed to ensure there is no rectal injury.

4. Further management should continue to be conservative if possible. After a period of approximately three months, ascending and descending urethrograms can be performed to assess the extent of any stricture (**3** and **4**). Operative intervention should be delayed until all inflammation has settled and the tissues are as normal as possible. If the patient is left with a narrow stricture, an optical urethrotomy may be successful. Urethral stents are generally contraindicated, so it is often necessary to proceed to open excision of the strictured area and urethroplasty. Larger urethral defects can be bridged by judicious use of pedicled penile or scrotal skin, as was necessary in this case (**5–8**).

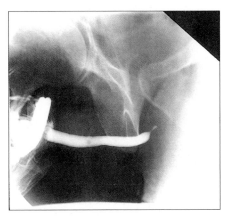

3 Ascending urethrogram showing residual stricture.

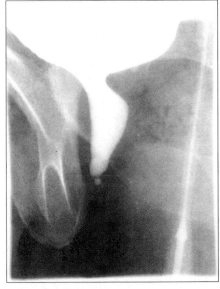

4 Descending urethrogram showing residual stricture.

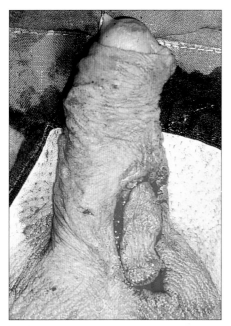

5 Reconstruction of urethra with isolation of skin graft.

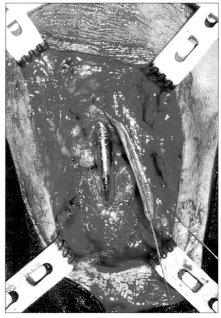

6 Extent of defect in urethra after apposition of anterior wall.

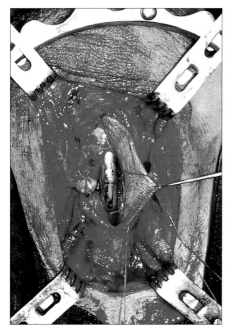

7 Skin graft being sutured to defect.

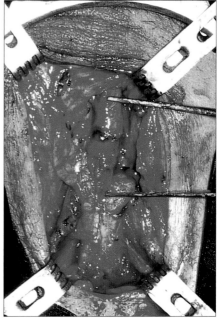

8 Final result.

Case 16
Complication of a Herniorraphy

A 46-year-old diabetic patient underwent a routine left inguinal herniorraphy and was discharged the following day. Two days later he was readmitted, having developed a pyrexia and become increasingly confused. On examination, there was marked scrotal swelling with palpable crepitus (1).

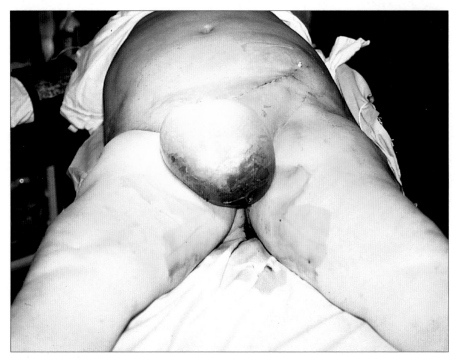

1 Appearance on presentation.

QUESTIONS
1. What is the diagnosis (1) and what is its cause?
2. What treatment is required?

ANSWERS

1. Synergistic necrotising fasciitis (Fournier's gangrene). There is no specific causative agent, but combined infection occurs with a variety of organisms such as *Bacteroides*, *Klebsiella*, *Proteus*, *Pseudomonas* and *Clostridium*.

2. Treatment consists of intravenous broad-spectrum antibiotics and urgent surgical debridement. Initial debridement consisted of excision of all scrotal skin (**2**) but, as is often the case, more extensive surgery was required due to the development of further gangrene. The extent of the debridement needed to excise all affected tissue is shown (**3**). Despite this aggressive management, mortality approaches 50%. Subsequently, plastic surgery was required to repair the defect, and in particular, to cover the testes (**4** and **5**).

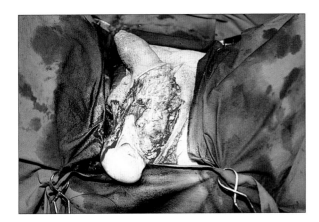

2 Extent of initial debridement.

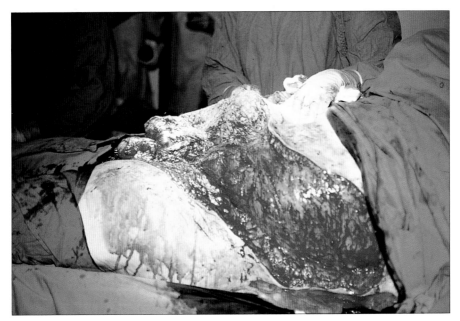

3 Extent of subsequent debridement.

Case 16

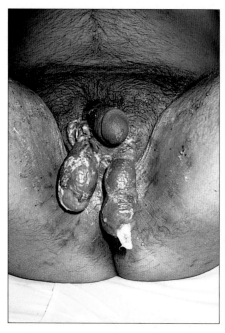

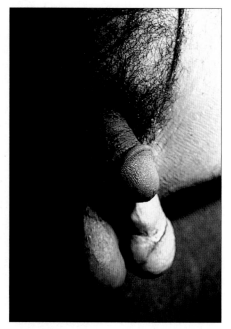

4 Split skin grafts applied to testes to replace lost scrotal skin.

5 Final result.

Case 17
Abdominal Pain and Hypertension

A 45-year-old woman presented with a six-week history of generalised abdominal discomfort. On examination, her blood pressure was raised at 170/105 mmHg. Her abdomen appeared to be distended, and on palpation both kidneys were easily palpable. There was no family history of renal disease. Urinalysis showed microscopic haematuria, and her serum electrolytes and creatinine were normal. An IVU (**1**) and ultrasound scan (**2**) were performed.

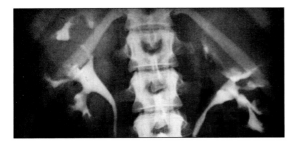

1 IVU at presentation. (Reprinted from Lloyd–Davies, W., Parkhouse, H., Gow, J. and Davies, D., *Color Atlas of Urology, Second Edition,* Wolfe Publishing, London, 1994.)

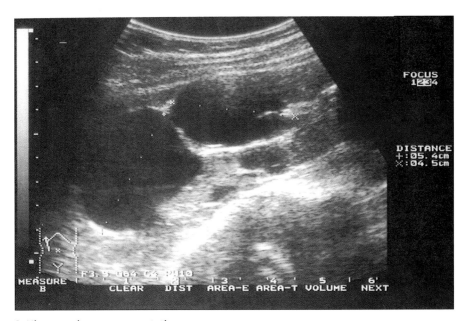

2 Ultrasound scan at presentation.

QUESTIONS
1. What is the likely diagnosis?
2. What associated conditions are there?
3. What complications may ensue, and how should they be managed?

Case 17

ANSWERS

1. The IVU shows large kidneys with bilateral distortion of the renal calyces. The likely diagnosis is, therefore, the adult type of polycystic kidney disease (PKD). This is inherited as an austosomal-dominant genetic condition, with the responsible gene located on chromosome 16.

2. PKD is associated with similar polycystic disease in the liver and pancreas. This may be confirmed by CT scan (**3**). There is a high incidence (up to 35%) of berry aneurysm, and thus a significant risk of subarachnoid haemorrhage. Associations of PKD with mitral valve prolapse and diverticular disease are also described.

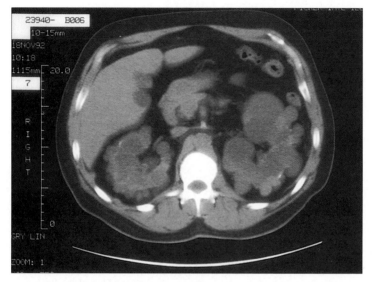

3 CT scan showing polycystic disease of kidneys, liver and pancreas.

3. Complications of PKD include urinary infections, pain, haematuria and renal failure. Infections should be treated with antibiotics as necessary. If there is severe pain, this may necessitate deroofing of the cysts (Rovsing's operation), although the benefit of this procedure is debatable. Nephrectomy should be avoided, if at all possible, because of the inevitability of renal failure; however, when this occurs, nephrectomy may be undertaken for symptomatic relief or to allow enough space for a renal transplant (**4**). In the meantime, dialysis will be required.

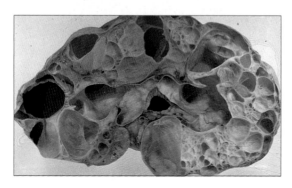

4 Nephrectomy specimen. (Reprinted from Lloyd–Davies, W., Parkhouse, H., Gow, J. and Davies, D., *Color Atlas of Urology, Second Edition*, Wolfe Publishing, London, 1994.)

Case 18
Urinary Tract Infection

A 61-year-old office worker presented with a three-month history of dysuria, weight loss and general malaise. Two urine samples had confirmed the presence of coliform organisms with pyuria and microscopic haematuria. Physical examination was normal.

QUESTIONS
1. What abnormalities are shown on the IVU (**1**)?
2. What is shown by the biopsy specimens (**2** and **3**, overleaf)?
3. How is this lesion staged?
4. How should this patient be treated?

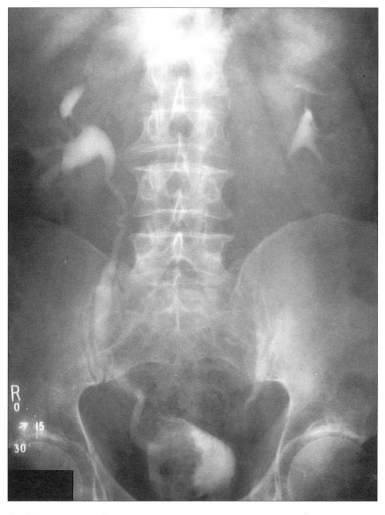

1 IVU at presentation.

Case 18

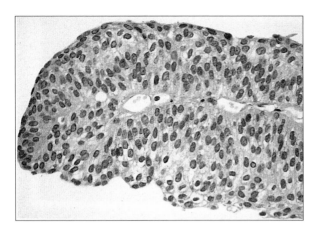

2 Biopsy.

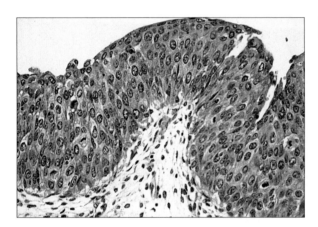

3 Additional bladder biopsy.

ANSWERS

1. There is a large filling defect in the right side of the bladder with a degree of ureteric obstruction. The likely diagnosis is a carcinoma of the bladder. This was confirmed through a cystoscopy, which revealed a single 5 cm-diameter semi-solid papillary lesion on the right bladder wall. After resection, there was no palpable mass on bimanual examination.

2. The histology shows a poorly differentiated transitional-cell carcinoma invading the muscularis propria but not advancing into the detrusor muscle itself. Carcinoma *in situ* is present in the additional biopsy.

3. Carcinoma of the bladder is staged according to the TNM system, as shown in **Table 1**. Pathologically, the tumour is defined according to cellular differentiation, which may be good (G1), moderate (G2) or poor (G3).

Table 1 TNM Classification of Bladder Carcinoma

TUMOUR	Carcinoma *in situ*	Tis
	Tumour superficial to muscularis mucosa	Ta
	Tumour invading muscularis mucosa	T1
	Tumour invading superficial bladder muscle	T2
	Deep invasion of bladder muscle	T3a
	Invasion into perivesical fat	T3b
	Involvement of prostate	T4a
	Involvement of other adjacent structures	T4b
NODES	Single positive node < 2 cm	N1
	Node or nodes < 5 cm	N2
	Larger nodes	N3
METASTASES		
	No metastases	M0
	Metastases	M1

4. This patient's tumour is superficial and poorly differentiated, and therefore should be staged as pT1 G3. These tumours are aggressive, and, if untreated, show a progression rate to invasion of 40% within three years. Immediate further treatment is therefore required.

Choice of treatment lies between further resections, a course of intravesical chemotherapy and radical surgery. Because of the additional area involved when carcinoma is *in situ*, this patient was treated with a six-week course of intravesical chemotherapy (BCG) and a further cystoscopy was performed two months later. No further tumour was seen, so the patient was kept under regular cystoscopic review, but unfortunately later defaulted.

Four years later, the patient represented complaining of haematuria, not having attended for 12 months previously. Cystoscopy showed a large posterior bladder tumour which, histologically, was moderately differentiated and invasive (pT3,G2) (**4**).

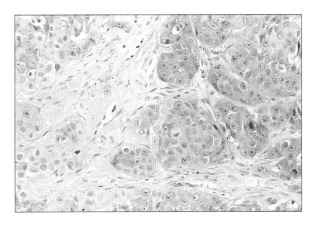

4 Bladder biopsy at re-presentation showing tumour invasion of deep muscle.

Case 18

QUESTION

5. What further treatment is indicated?

ANSWER

5. The patient should undergo a radical cystoprostatectomy (**5**). In the presence of carcinoma *in situ*, a urethrectomy and ileal loop diversion is usually indicated. However, this patient was keen to preserve his bladder if possible. As his prostate biopsies were normal, he therefore underwent a reconstruction using a folded loop of ileum (**6–12**) to create the neobladder which was then anastamosed to the membranous urethra. Subsequent check urethroscopies are planned as the risk of a urethral tumour recurrence in his case is approximately 10%.

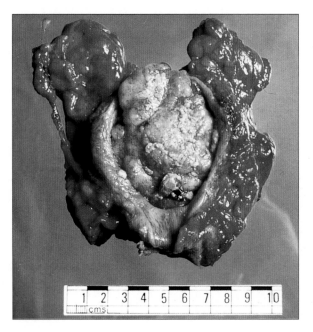

5 Macroscopic appearance of cystectomy specimen.

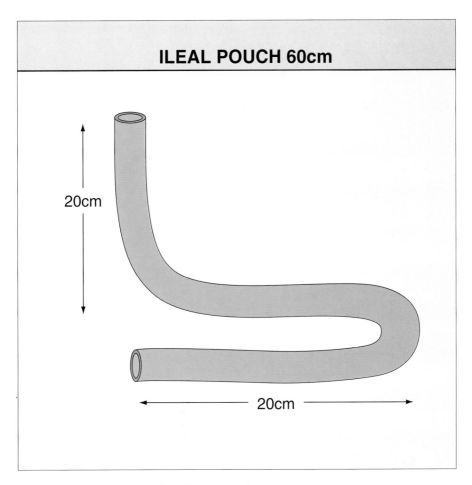

ILEAL POUCH 60cm

20cm

20cm

6 Diagrammatic representation of reconstruction.

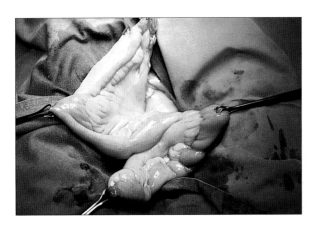

7 Ileal segments for use in reconstruction.

Case 18

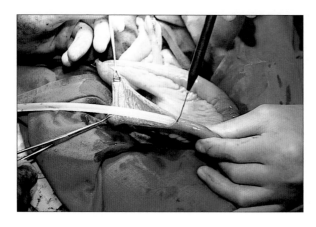

8 Opening ileum along antimesenteric border.

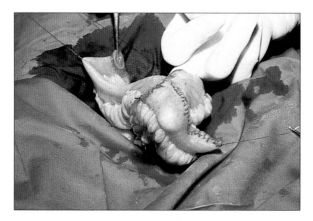

9 Completed neobladder with afferent ileal loop. The inserted finger marks the site for anastamosis to the urethra.

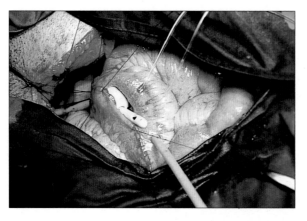

10 Suprapubic and urethral catheters in position. The first urethral suture can be seen.

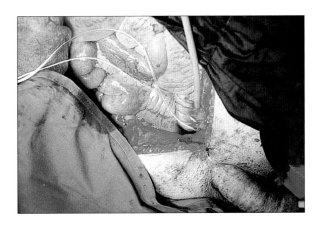

11 Completed anastamosis. The ureteric stents are seen.

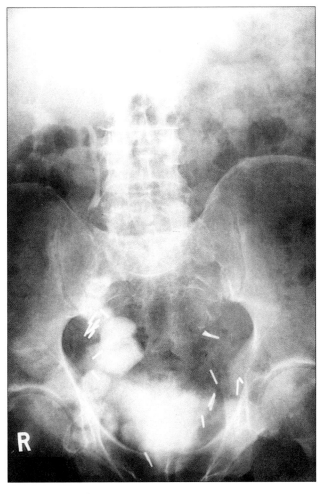

12 Post-operative IVU.

Case 19

An Accident in the Playground

A 7-year-old boy fell off a climbing frame on to his back from a distance of two feet above the ground. He did not complain of pain at the time of the injury, and there was no evidence of external bruising. One hour later, however, he complained of severe abdominal pain, and was noted to have a very distended abdomen. He was able to pass urine without difficulty, but had frank haematuria.

QUESTIONS
1. How should this child be managed initially?
2. What do the initial imaging investigations show (1– 4)?
3. How do these investigations influence management?
4. How should this child be managed in the long term?

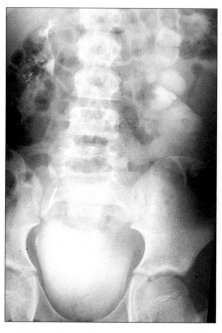

1 IVU performed in Accident and Emergency Department.

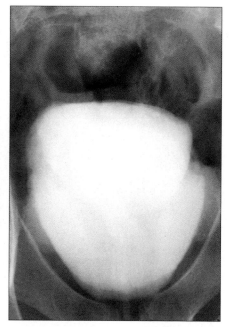

2 Post-micturition film of IVU.

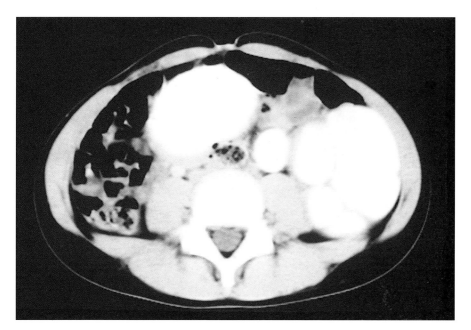

3 CT of abdomen.

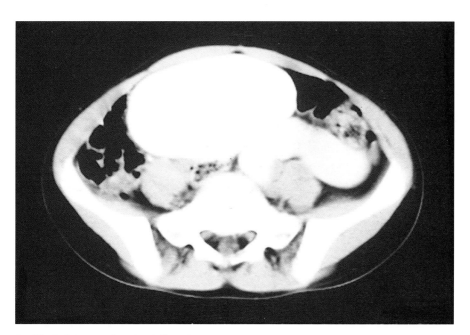

4 CT of abdomen showing left ureter.

Case 19

ANSWERS

1. In view of the relatively trivial nature of the injury and the absence of external bruising or bony injury, a congenital abnormality of the urinary tract should be suspected. Resuscitation, if necessary, is the first priority, and careful monitoring of pulse, blood pressure and urine output is essential. If the patient is haemodynamically stable, with no evidence of peritonism, there is no indication for immediate surgical intervention. Urgent radiological imaging of the urinary tract should be carried out.

2. The IVU (**1**) showed hydronephrotic left kidney with possible extravasation of contrast medium. No bony or other soft tissue injuries are evident. Post-micturition film of the bladder shows a large-capacity bladder which empties poorly (**2**). A CT scan was done while the IV contrast medium was still in the urinary tract (**3, 4**), and shows left-sided hydro-ureteronephrosis with no evidence of extravasation, consistent with a diagnosis of mega-ureter.

3. As the imaging has excluded a major urological injury, conservative treatment is favoured, unless there is a change in the patient's clinical condition. In view of the large-capacity, poorly emptying bladder, a micturating cysto-urethrogram was performed to look for vesico-ureteric reflux and urethral abnormalities (**5**). The micturating cysto-urethrogram shows a normal urethra with no evidence of vesico-ureteric reflux.

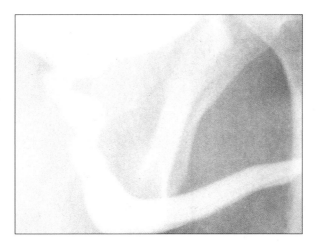

5 Micturating cysto-urethrogram.

4. A Tc^{99m} myelin-associated glycoprotein (MAG) 3 renogram two months after the injury (**6**) showed normal function on the affected side with slow drainage after administration of frusemide, consistent with stasis rather than obstruction. A decision was made to perform a ureteric reimplant, with plication of the mega-ureter, rather than nephrectomy. This decision resulted in preservation of renal function, as renography two years after surgery shows no appreciable change in differential function, although drainage from the left kidney is still sluggish (**7**).

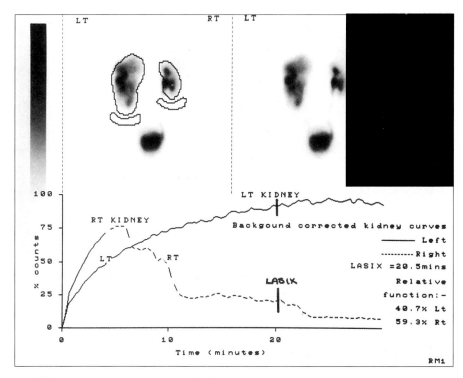

6 Tc[99m] MAG 3 renogram two months after injury.

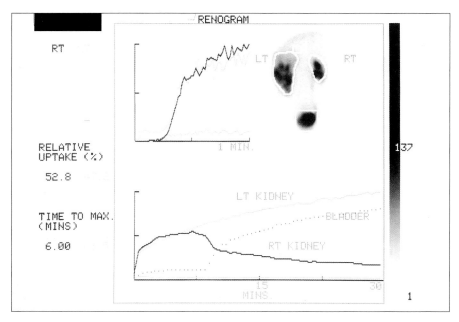

7 Tc[99m] diethylenetriamine penta-acetic acid (DTPA) renogram two years after re-implantation of left ureter.

67

Case 20
Urinary Tract Infection after Sexual Intercourse

A 30-year-old lady who had been married for three years complained of severe dysuria and rigors on every occasion after sexual intercourse with her husband. This was so severe that it had resulted in complete abstinence from sexual activity for over one year. Prophylactic antibiotics had not helped to alleviate her symptoms. She had no significant past medical history.

QUESTIONS

1. What do the ultrasound scans of the right (**1**) and left (**2**) kidneys show?
2. What further investigation is indicated, and what does this show?
3. What further steps should be taken to establish a diagnosis?
4. What further radiological investigation is indicated, and how should management then proceed?

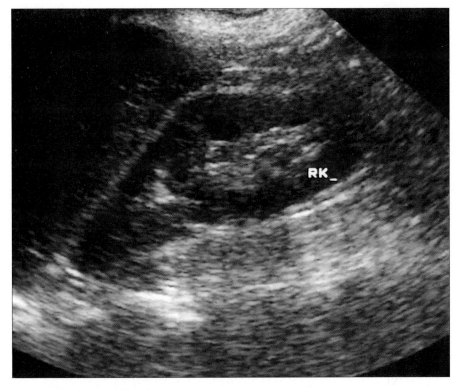

1 Ultrasound scan of right kidney.

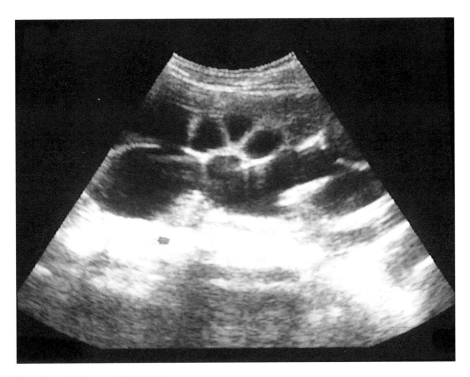

2 Ultrasound scan of left kidney.

ANSWERS

1. The ultrasound scan of the right kidney (**1**) shows a possible duplex system with no evidence of hydronephrosis. The scan of the left kidney (**2**) shows a cystic structure at the upper pole.

2. The IVU is indicated to show renal anatomy (**3** and **4**). This shows a duplex system on the right side, and a lower pole moiety of a possible duplex system on the left (**3**). However, no function is seen in the upper pole. The bladder empties well following micturition, but there is some residual contrast medium in the lower left ureter, which is dilated, indicating the possibility of vesico-ureteric reflux, or lower ureteric obstruction. A micturating cysto-urethrogram failed to demonstrate vesico-ureteric reflux on either side.

Case 20

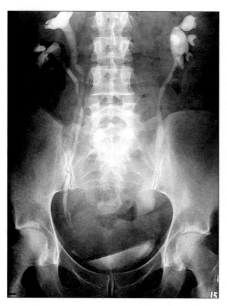

3 IVU.

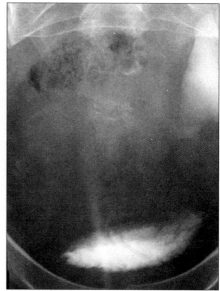

4 Post-micturition film of IVU.

3. In view of the cystic lesion at the left upper pole, this must be assumed to be a non-functioning upper pole moiety until proved otherwise. Cystoscopy and retrograde ureterography may help in outlining the anatomy. At cystoscopy, a single ureteric orifice was seen on either side, and no ectopic orifices were seen in the bladder or vagina. A retrograde ureteric catheter was inserted into the left ureter, and further imaging was done in the X–ray Department (**5**). The retrograde ureterogram shows a single ureter with the previously noted lower pole moiety demonstrated, corresponding to the IVU appearance. However, the radiologist has left the retrograde catheter *in situ* as far as the renal pelvis. Without withdrawing the ureteric catheter and reinjecting contrast medium, it is impossible to rule out a second ureter with a low insertion into the lower pole ureter.

4. As there is strong suspicion of a left duplex system, an antegrade study is indicated. The left upper pole cystic swelling was punctured under ultrasound guidance and contrast was introduced (**6** and **7**). This investigation clearly shows a grossly dilated upper pole moiety with a mega-ureter and a low insertion into the lower pole ureter. The patient was treated with an upper pole heminephro-ureterectomy with complete resolution of her symptoms, which delighted both her and her husband.

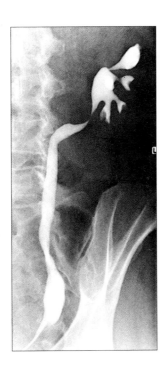

5 Left retrograde ureterogram.

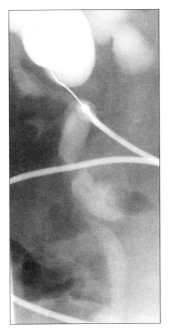

6 Left antegrade pyelo-ureterogram.

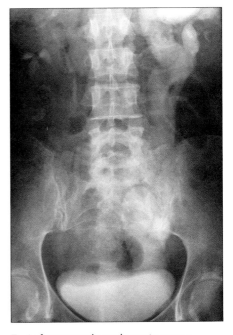

7 Left antegrade pyelo-ureterogram.

A Man With Renal Failure

A 65-year-old man who did not speak English presented with acute renal failure. He was known to have had major surgery in early childhood. Inspection of his genitalia provided a clue to his previous history (1). He also carried with him some radiographs which had been taken several years previously, one of which is shown in 2. An ultrasound scan of the urinary tract showed a small scarred right kidney and a hydronephrotic left kidney with good cortical thickness. The bladder could not be demonstrated.

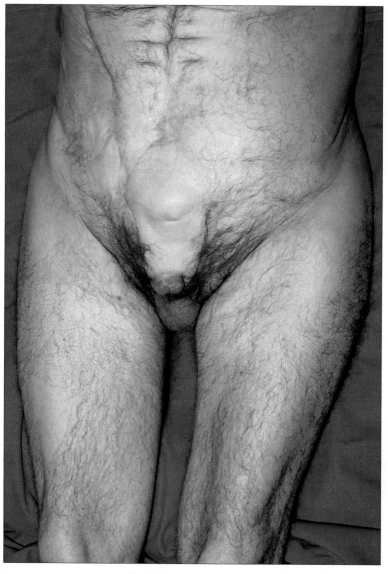

1 Appearance of external genitalia.

Case 21

QUESTIONS
1. What is the diagnosis, based on examination of his genitalia (**1**)?
2. What does the radiograph show (**2**)?
3. What is the most likely cause for his renal failure?
4. What does the sigmoid colon biopsy show (**3**)?
5. How should this situation be managed?

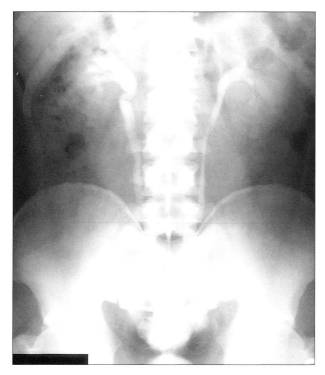

2 Radiograph.

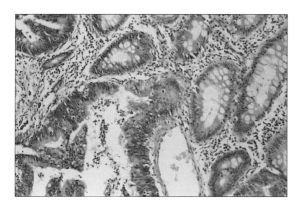

3 Histology of sigmoid colon biopsy.

Case 21

ANSWERS

1. There is no pubic hair in the midline, and the pubic bones are widely separated. There is evidence of previous genital surgery. It is possible that this man was born with bladder extrophy.
2. This is an IVU showing bilateral functioning kidneys, both of which drain into the bowel. It is likely that this man had a cystectomy in childhood, with urinary diversion by means of bilateral ureterosigmoidostomies.
3. The most likely cause of the renal failure is chronic obstruction to the right ureter with acute obstruction to the left ureter. In view of the history of uretero-sigmoidostomies, the most likely pathology is a tumour at the junction of the ureters and bowel. This was confirmed on sigmoidoscopy and biopsy (**3**).
4. The histology shows adenocarcinoma of sigmoid colon (**3**). These tumours commonly occur at the junction of the ureters and bowel when there has been a mixing of the urinary and faecal streams for many years.
5. The acute renal failure was managed with immediate decompression of the left kidney by percutaneous nephrostomy. Following the return of the renal function to normal, the urinary diversion was converted to an ileal conduit, and an anterior resection of the bowel tumour was carried out. As the man was potent and wished to maintain his potency, bladder reconstruction was not attempted. Pathological staging of the bowel tumour was Duke's stage B.

Case 22
A Young Woman in Retention

A 30-year-old woman presented to the Accident and Emergency Department with sudden onset of complete urinary retention, but with no significant past medical history (1 and 2). She was catheterised and admitted to hospital.

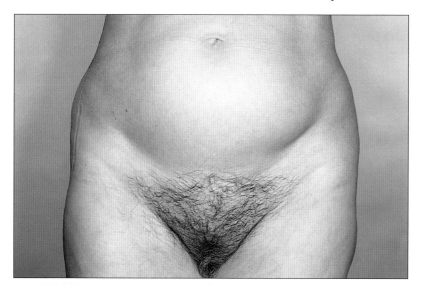

1 Abdomen of woman in retention.

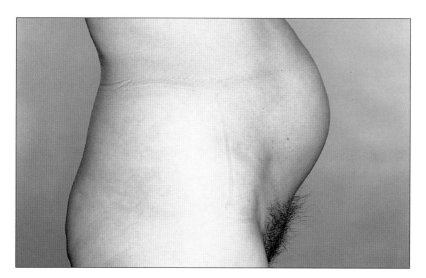

2 Lateral view of abdomen.

QUESTIONS
1. How should this situation be managed?
2. What investigations may be helpful?
3. What is the treatment for this condition?

Case 22

1. It is important to exclude obvious causes for retention such as pelvic pathology, medication and constipation. An ultrasound of the urinary tract and pelvis revealed no abnormalities in this case.
2. Urethral sphincter electromyogram (EMG) with analysis of individual motor units may be helpful in demonstrating abnormalities due to re-innervation (**3**), when the motor units are obviously different from normal (**4**). This pattern may be associated with the polycystic ovarian syndrome, but full neurological assessment should also be carried out in order to exclude conditions such as multiple sclerosis. Some psychiatric conditions may also present in this way.

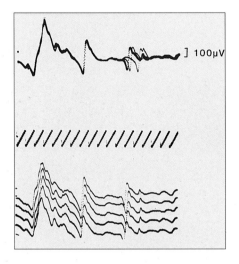

3 Abnormal EMG recording of individual motor unit.

] 100µV

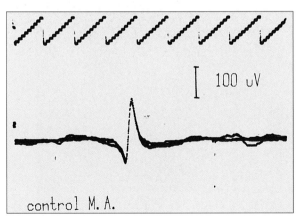

4 Normal EMG recording of individual motor unit.

3. Acute retention in young women with no obvious cause can be very difficult to treat. Drugs which relax the urethral sphincter, such as alpha blockers, are occasionally helpful, but often, intermittent self-catheterisation is the only way to manage these patients until normal voiding is established. This often takes many months.

Case 23
Jogger's Haematuria

A 30-year-old marathon runner complained of heavy haematuria after strenuous exercise, but he was otherwise well. His blood pressure was normal, and flexible cystoscopy revealed no bladder abnormalities.

QUESTIONS
1. What do the plain film of the right kidney (**1**) and IVU (**2**) show?
2. How should this be managed?
3. How should he be followed up after treatment?
4. What does the Tc^{99m}DTPA renogram show (**3**)?

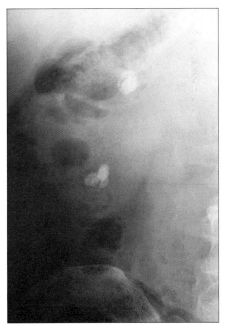

1 Plain film of right kidney.

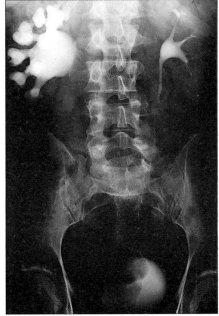

3 Tc^{99m}DTPA renogram.

2 IVU.

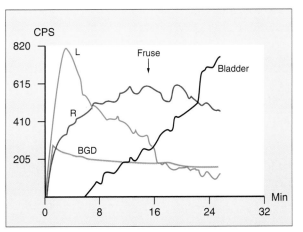

Case 23

ANSWERS

1. The plain film shows several opacities within the right kidney (**1**). After IV contrast (**2**), a dilated right pelvi-calyceal system is seen, consistent with a diagnosis of pelvi-ureteric junction obstruction. The right ureter is not demonstrated.
2. The stones were treated initially with lithotripsy, after inserting a double pigtail stent. **4** shows a plain film after successful disintegration of the lower pole stones. Following clearance of the upper pole stone, the double pigtail stent was removed. Metabolic studies showed no obvious primary aetiology for the stone.

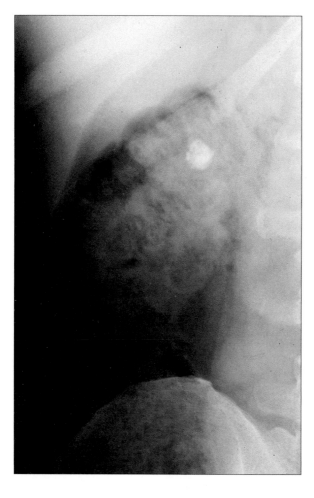

4 Plain film of right kidney.

3. It is important to establish whether pelvi-ureteric junction obstruction is persistent after stone disintegration. This can be done with a $Tc^{99m}DTPA$ renogram (**3**).
4. The renogram shows persistent obstruction to the right kidney (**3**); the correct treatment for this is pyeloplasty.

Case 24
An Infant with a Possible Immunological Deficiency

A one-year-old boy having an older brother with known auto-immune disease presented with fever. His mother had a lesion on the trunk, which was diagnosed as herpes zoster (1). The boy was assumed to have an auto-immune disorder, and was admitted to hospital for barrier nursing. Extensive serological investigations failed to show any abnormalities, but MSU showed a significant growth of *Escherichia coli*. A plain abdominal radiographical examination was performed (2).

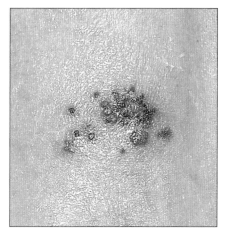

1 Skin lesion on trunk of boy's mother.

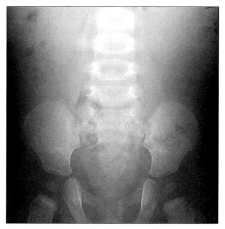

2 Plain abdominal radiograph.

QUESTIONS
1. What does the plain abdominal radiograph show (2)?
2. What does the CT scan show (3)?
3. What further radiological investigation is appropriate?
4. How should this be managed?

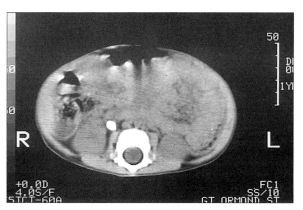

3 CT scan of abdomen.

Case 24

ANSWERS

1. A small area of calcification in the right side of the abdomen (2). This was assumed to be in the inferior vena cava, so a CT scan of the abdomen was performed (3).
2. The CT without IV contrast shows that there is a calcific lesion in the line of the ureter (3).
3. As there is strong possibility of a ureteric stone, an IVU should be performed (4 and 5). This shows an impacted ureteric stone with an obstructed right kidney.
4. This was treated with open ureterolithotomy under antibiotic cover, as the child was too small and too ill for minimally invasive techniques. He made a swift recovery following stone removal, and metabolic studies revealed no obvious underlying aetiology for the stone. He did, however, suffer with recurrent balanitis, and circumcision was recommended.

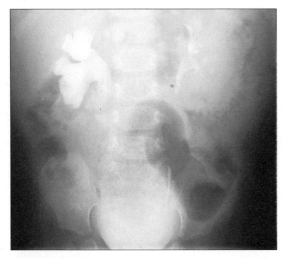

4 IVU.

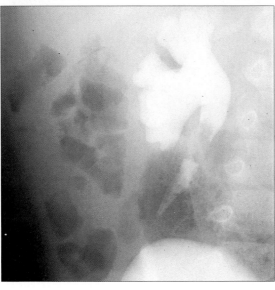

5 IVU (oblique view).

Case 25

A Peculiar Swelling

A 34-year-old man presented with a two-year history of a gradually enlarging swelling on his scrotum which had recently started discharging a small amount of yellowish fluid. On examination, there was a 4×1 cm firm swelling hanging from the right side of his scrotum, with ulceration of the skin at its lower end (**1** and **2**). It was not attached to the scrotal contents. The lesion was excised under local anaesthetic.

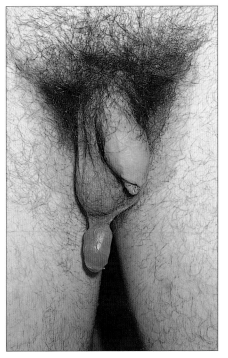

1 Appearance on presentation.

2 Appearance on presentation.

QUESTION
1. What does the histology show (**3**), and what is the diagnosis?

3 Histological appearance.

Case 25

ANSWER

1. The histology (**3**) shows interweaving bundles of eosinophilic cells, strongly suggestive of smooth muscle. It is likely that the tumour has in fact arisen in the dartos muscle. The mitotic index is low; therefore the likely diagnosis is of a leiomyoma.

   Leiomyomas of the skin are rare, and may occur on the scrotum or labia. Histologically, they are similar to piloleiomyomas. This lesion is similar to the scalp lesion described by Edward Cock, and is sometimes known as Cock's peculiar tumour.

Case 26
Impotence

A 48-year-old man presented with a 12-month history of loss of erections. Two years previously he had divorced, and he now wished to remarry. Four years previously he had undergone coronary artery bypass grafting, from which he made a complete recovery. He was not taking any drugs. Physical examination was normal. Initial investigations revealed normal blood glucose, serum testosterone and prolactin levels.

QUESTION
1. What further investigations and treatments are appropriate?

ANSWER
1. From the history, it is not clear whether this man's impotence is caused by organic or psychological factors. An intracavernosal injection of a vaso-active agent such as papaverine or prostaglandin E1 should be administered, and if an erection ensues, the patient should be taught the technique of self-injection (**1–3**). Prostaglandin E1 has a lower risk of inducing a prolonged erection, and is therefore the drug of choice. If the impotence is of psychogenic origin, there is a 25% chance that spontaneous erections will resume with time.

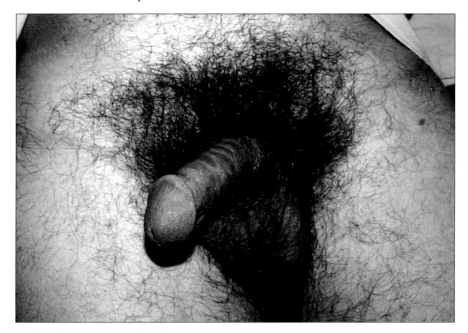

1 Flaccid penis prior to injection.

Case 26

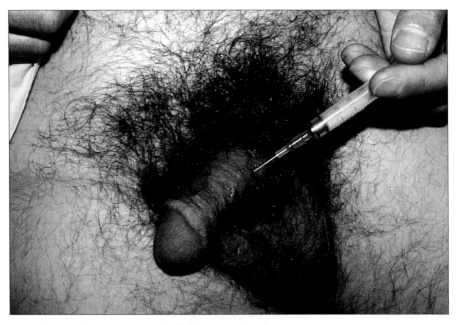

2 Technique of intracavernosal self-injection.

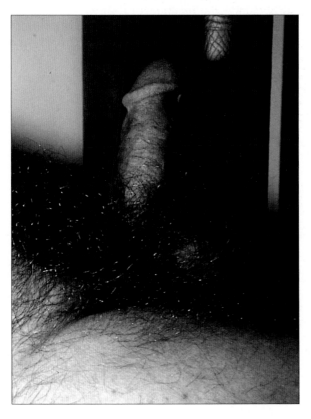

3 Result of intracavernosal self-injection.

Case 26

If he fails to respond to intracavernosal injections, there may be a vascular cause for the erectile failure. It is then appropriate to perform a colour duplex scan of the penile arteries (**4** and **5**) and a cavernosogram (**6** and **7**). If these show significant vascular abnormalities, corrective surgery may be possible. If not, the patient is best treated by insertion of a penile prosthesis.

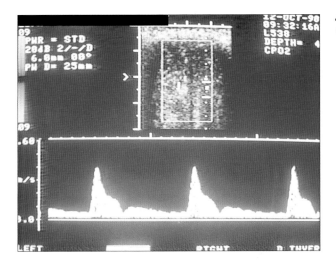

4 Colour duplex scan of normal penile vessels.

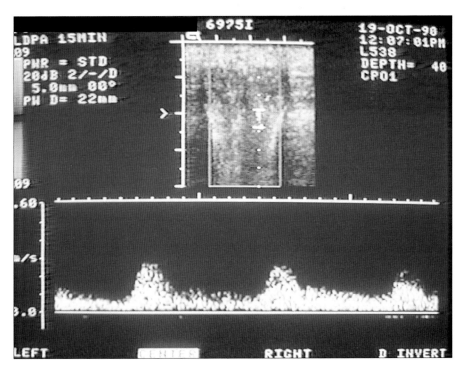

5 Colour duplex scan in arterial impotence.

Case 26

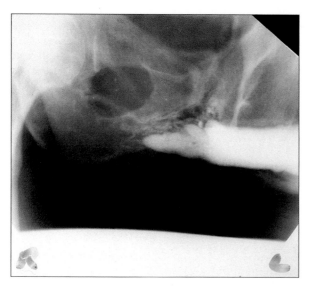

6 Normal cavernosogram.

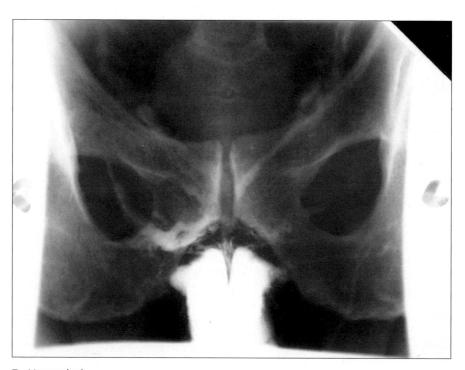

7 Venous leak.

Case 27

Bilateral Testicular Swellings

A 70-year-old man presented with a six-week history of increasing discomfort and swelling of both testicles. There was no history of trauma and he denied any other urinary tract symptoms. His health was generally good, although he did admit to weight loss of approximately seven pounds over the preceding two months.

On examination, there were bilateral testicular swellings (1). The remainder of his abdomen was soft, and on general examination there were no other abnormal features. An ultrasound scan of his scrotum was undertaken (2).

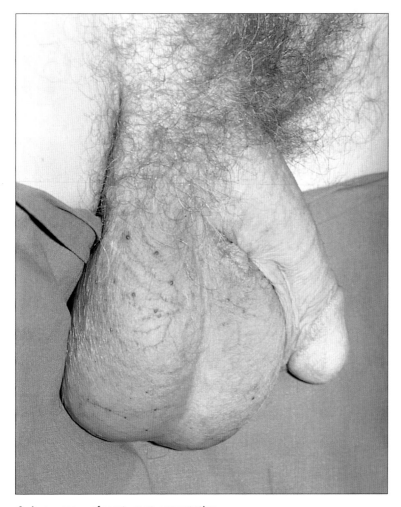

1 Appearance of scrotum at presentation.

Case 27

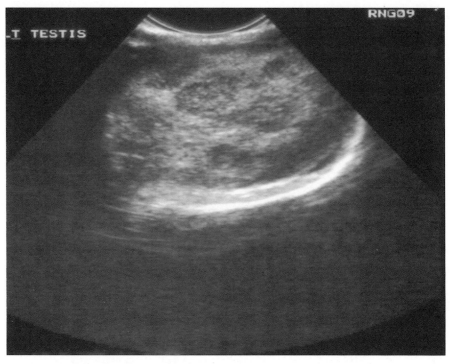

2 Ultrasound scan of testis at presentation.

QUESTIONS
1. What is the likely diagnosis?
2. What further investigations and treatment are required?

ANSWERS

1. The ultrasound scan shows a solid testicular swelling. In a man aged 70 the most likely diagnosis is therefore testicular lymphoma although other possibilities including teratoma, seminoma or a mixed testicular tumour must be considered.
2. A chest radiograph should be performed and blood should be taken for the tumour markers AFP and beta human chorionic gonadotrophin. In this case, though, the values of both these markers were normal. Tissue should then be obtained for histological examination. This patient underwent an orchidectomy in the right testis, since it was the most painful of his testes (**3** and **4**). The left testis was not removed so as to act as a marker lesion to monitor the progress of subsequent treatment.

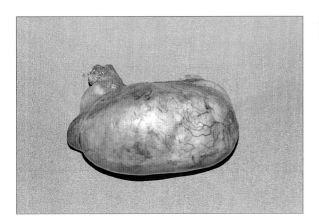

3 Operative appearance of right testis.

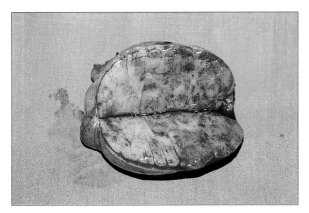

4 Section through right testis.

Histology of the testis showed a B-cell lymphoma (**5**). CT scans were therefore undertaken of the chest, abdomen and pelvis, and para-aortic lymphadenopathy was detected (**6**). The patient was commenced on a course of systemic chemotherapy consisting of cyclophosphamide, donorubicin, vincristine and prednisolone (CHOP); a subsequent decrease in size of the left testis confirmed a good response to treatment.

Case 27

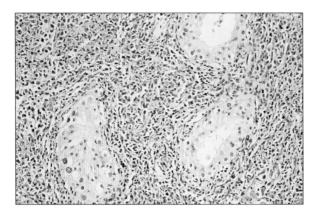

5 Histological appearance showing B-cell lymphoma.

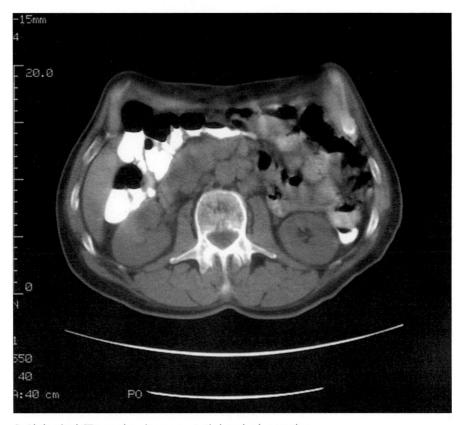

6 Abdominal CT scan showing para-aortic lymphadenopathy.

Index

Index